Handbook of Endometrial Pathology

Debra S Heller
Professor of Pathology and Laboratory Medicine
Joint Professor of Obstetrics, Gynecology and Women's Health
University of Medicine and Dentistry of New Jersey, Newark, USA

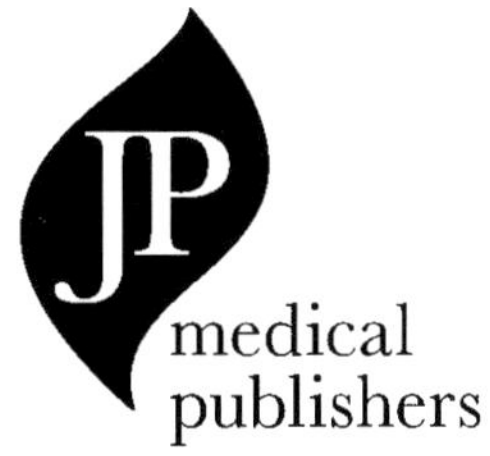

London • Panama City • New Delhi

© 2012 JP Medical Ltd.
Published by JP Medical Ltd,
83 Victoria Street, London, SW1H 0HW, UK
Tel: +44 (0)20 3170 8910
Fax: +44 (0)20 3008 6180
Email: info@jpmedpub.com
Web: www.jpmedpub.com

ISBN: 978-1-907816-10-9

British Library Cataloguing in Publication Data
A catalogue record for this book is available from the British Library

Library of Congress Cataloging in Publication Data
A catalog record for this book is available from the Library of Congress

JP Medical Ltd is a subsidiary of Jaypee Brothers Medical Publishers (P) Ltd, New Delhi, India

Publisher: Geoff Greenwood
Editorial Assistant: Katrina Rimmer
Design: Designers Collective Ltd

Typeset, printed and bound in India.

Preface

Endometrial biopsy specimens are among the most frequent specimens crossing the pathologist's bench, and among the most complicated. The clinical picture, including such information as patient's age, hormonal interventions, and menstrual status, are often critical to the interpretation of the specimen, and yet may not be provided. There are many artifacts that interfere with interpretation as well. Nevertheless, the clinician expects a short, comprehensible report that can guide management and be explained to the patient.

This book provides the practicing pathologist with the tools to improve diagnostic accuracy of endometrial biopsy specimens, while providing insight to the clinician caring for women. By imparting an understanding of the clinical aspects, as well as the potential histopathological difficulties, it is hoped that the goal of the best patient care is achieved.

Debra S Heller
February 2012

Contents

Dedication

To all the good men. Without them there could be no good women.

Abbreviations

APA	atypical polypoid adenomyoma
bhCG	beta human chorionic gonadotropin
CEA	carcinoembryonic antigen
CK-18	cytokeratin-18
COX-2	cyclo-oxygenase-2
DUB	dysfunctional uterine bleeding
EIC	endometrial intraepithelial carcinoma
EIN	endometrial intraepithelial neoplasia
ER/PR	estrogen and progesterone receptor
ESS	endometrial stromal sarcoma
ETT	epithelioid trophoblastic tumor
FIGO	International Federation of Gynecology and Obstetrics
FISH	fluorescent in situ hybridization
GTD	gestational trophoblastic disease
GTN	gestational trophoblastic neoplasia
H&E	hematoxylin and eosin
hCG	human chorionic gonadotropin
Her2/neu	human epidermal growth factor receptor 2
hPL	human placental lactogen
HPV	human papilloma virus
HRT	hormone replacement therapy
IMP3	insulin-like growth factor II messenger RNA binding protein-3
LEEP	loop electrosurgical excision procedure
LVSI	lymphovascular space involvement
Mel-CAM	CD146 (also mel-cell adhesion molecule)
MMP	matrix metalloproteinase
PAX2	paired box gene 2
POD	postovulatory day
PSTT	placental site trophoblastic tumor
PTEN	phosphatase and tensin homologue
PVA	polyvinyl alcohol particles
TCC	transitional cell carcinoma
VPS	volume percent stroma
WHO	World Health Organization

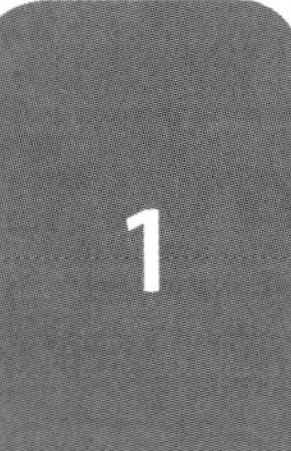

Interpreting pathology results – the value of communication

Introduction

Pathology interpretations are not always black and white, and shades of grey are common. For optimal patient care, it is essential that the women's health clinician and the pathologist understand each other and communicate. Clinical information is essential to the pathologist for formulating an appropriate diagnosis or differential diagnosis, and such information does not prejudice the interpretation. The pathologist needs to know whether patients have been given hormonal medications to control bleeding prior to sampling, or are on oral contraceptives, hormone replacement therapy, tamoxifen, or other hormonal medications: these all have effects on endometrial morphology. Age, menopausal status, pertinent prior surgery, and any other contributory history are also important. In turn, pathologists need to provide a report that is interpretable and clinically useful. The following discussion is provided to assist each specialty in understanding the other.

Some gynecology for the pathologist

Why is endometrial sampling performed?

There are a number of reasons. Endometrial sampling is most often performed for abnormal uterine bleeding. As part of the evaluation of infertility, it has fallen in popularity with the availability of more accurate serological tests of hormonal status. It may be warranted by a thickened endometrial stripe on transvaginal ultrasound, particularly in a postmenopausal woman. A biopsy may be performed to monitor therapy for hyperplasia, or if there is any suspicion of or a need to rule out malignancy, such as abnormal endometrial cells on a pap smear.

Abnormal bleeding may be categorized as shown in **Table 1.1**. In the reproductive age group, pregnancy-related causes of bleeding, including intrauterine pregnancy, ectopic pregnancy, and gestational trophoblastic disease, must always be considered. Rarely, systemic disease, such as a coagulation disorder, is the cause of abnormal uterine bleeding. Sometimes bleeding perceived as uterine by the patient is actually not of endometrial origin, or may even be nongenital, originating from the cervix, vagina, bladder, or rectum.

Table 1.1 Etiology of abnormal uterine bleeding

Etiology of abnormal uterine bleeding
Pregnancy-related
Iatrogenic
Systemic disease
Organic
Dysfunctional
Neoplasia

The more common etiologies in the peri- and postmenopausal woman are organic, dysfunctional and neoplastic etiologies. Organic causes of abnormal bleeding are lesions intrinsic to the uterus, such as submucous leiomyomas, adenomyosis or polyps. Abnormalities of angiogenesis are currently thought to be related to the bleeding seen with these lesions.[1–3] Dysfunctional uterine bleeding is abnormal bleeding in the absence of intrinsic uterine disease, pregnancy, systemic disease, or neoplasia, and is due to hormonal irregularities. Neoplasia may be hormonally related, or hormone-independent.

Depending on the bleeding pattern and age of the patient, an endometrial biopsy or curettage may be performed as part of the evaluation of the abnormal bleeding. Postmenopausal bleeding, although often due to atrophy, must always be investigated to rule out cancer, and this often necessitates endometrial sampling. This is discussed in more detail in subsequent chapters. Other techniques employed may include transvaginal ultrasound for assessment of thickness of the endometrium. A saline sonohysterogram may be a useful adjunct to transvaginal ultrasound, as the distention of the endometrial cavity separates the anterior and posterior walls, allowing for better identification of focal lesions such as polyps. Hysteroscopy, either in office or in the hospital, allows viewing of the cavity directly as well as allowing targeted sampling.

How is endometrial sampling performed?

In-office endometrial biopsy

Due to cost and convenience, in-office endometrial sampling is often the first modality utilized when endometrial sampling is undertaken. It is usually well-tolerated by the patient, as cervical dilatation is generally not necessary. Most of the current devices available are thin plastic catheters with an internal piston that creates suction, and an opening along the catheter to allow a scraping motion and collection of tissue, such as the Pipelle device. Such devices produce a plug of tissue, or blood admixed with tissue, which can be extruded into fixative and sent for histopathological evaluation.

There have been multiple studies on the accuracy of in-office devices in the sampling of the endometrium. In general, the devices sample less endometrium than does the curettage, but they are accurate for diffuse lesions, although focal lesions such as polyps may be missed.[4] Huang et al[5] found a sensitivity of 93.8% for Pipelle and 97% for curettage for low-grade cancers, and 99.2% and 100% respectively for high-grade cancers as compared with the pathology found at final hysterectomy. Although an older study showed that a much smaller percentage of the endometrium was sampled with a Pipelle compared to a Vabra aspirator,[6] in a more recent meta-analysis, the Pipelle was found to be more accurate than the Novak curette, Vabra aspirator, and a variety of lavage or cytological methods of sampling.[7] Some authors report success with a Tao brush, particularly in postmenopausal women. This modality provides a cytologic rather than histologic specimen,[8] however cytological endometrial sampling has not caught on in all locations. Because not all pathology laboratories may have experience evaluating cytologic endometrial specimens, discussion with the pathologist in advance of submitting such a specimen should be considered, as in any undertaking of a new method of evaluation.

Endometrial curettage

Often considered the "gold standard", cervical dilatation and endometrial curettage with a sharp curette provides more tissue for evaluation. However it requires anesthesia and is usually performed in a hospital or (often) an ambulatory care setting, hence it increases cost.

Some pathology for the clinician

Why is a history so important?

In years past, in the USA, trainees in obstetrics and gynecology often had the opportunity to rotate through the Pathology Department of their institution during training. With the mandatory hour restrictions in training programs, this exposure has become a great deal less frequent, and so clinicians may not have a sense of how pathology works or sufficient understanding of how important a history is in making a determination. Rarely do specimens look exactly like what is in the textbooks, and the rendering of a diagnosis is often a process of developing a differential diagnosis. Lack of clinical information impedes this, and may lead to a long descriptive diagnosis rather than a concise one. As an example, the diagnoses below are both from the same specimen. In the first case, no history of exogenous progesterone therapy was provided, and in the second it was:

- Diagnosis 1 (in the absence of history): endometrial tissue irregularly developed. The glands are small and inactive. The stroma is hypercellular and focally decidualized. This may represent exogenous progestational effect. Clinical correlation suggested.
- Diagnosis 2 (with history): benign endometrium, with glandular and stromal features consistent with progestin effect.

How does the pathologist evaluate tissue?

Gross Evaluation

Tissue is first examined grossly (by eye), and described in the report. The description generally includes whether the tissue was received fresh or in fixative, and the appearance of the tissue, including weight (for hysterectomies), size of the tissue or measurement in aggregate (for endometrial sampling), and appearance of the tissue. This is useful in cases where there is a discrepancy in the amount of tissue the clinician thinks was obtained, and what is seen on the slide. In some endometrial samples, most of what is in the device is actually blood, and this may give the clinician a false impression of abundant tissue. If the contents are ejected into formalin, this plug of tissue and blood may hold its shape, making it appear as though more tissue is there than is actually present. Rarely, tiny pieces of tissue either do not make it from the sampling device to the jar or get lost in processing in the pathology laboratory; the gross description can provide useful information here for comparison.

For larger resections, the gross description may give the distance of a visible tumor from margins, and the number, size, and character of any dissected lymph nodes for cancer procedures. If a microscopic assessment of margin status will be needed, ink may be applied to the specimen, so that the margins can be appreciated microscopically. This should all be reflected in the *gross description* portion of the pathology report.

The summary of sections lists what tissue was submitted to make the slides. In the case of a biopsy, generally all of the tissue is submitted, and is so stated. In a larger resection, submission of all the tissue is not practical, and representative sections are submitted. The summary of sections localizes the slides to where the tissue was taken from.

A typical gross description of an endometrial biopsy and a hysterectomy for uterine leiomyomata are given in the boxes below:

Typical gross description: **endometrial biopsy**

The specimen is labeled "endometrial curettings". Received fresh and consists of multiple fragments of pink/tan soft tissue admixed with blood clots measuring 2 cm × 1.9 cm × 0.8 cm in aggregate. The specimen is entirely submitted in one (1) cassette.

Typical gross description: **uterine leiomyomata**

The specimen is labeled, "Uterus and Cervix". Received in formalin is a uterus with attached cervix, weighing 150 g. The uterus measures 8 × 5 × 5 cm in width, length, and anterior to posterior. The external surface is smooth. The shape of the uterus is distorted by multiple nodules on the serosal surface, measuring 0.5–1.5 cm in greatest dimension. The cervix measures 3 × 3 cm in length and width. The exocervical mucosa is smooth. The os is patent, measuring 0.6 cm in diameter. Opening the specimen reveals an unremarkable transformation zone. The uterine cavity measures 4 × 1.5 cm, with a distorted shape. The endometrium, measuring 0.1 cm in thickness, is tan/brown. No polyp or focal lesion is identified. There are multiple nodules in the myometrium ranging in size from 0.6 to 3.6 cm in greatest dimension. The cut surfaces are tan/white with a whorled appearance. They are located subserosally and intramurally. The thickness of the myometrium measures 1.4 cm at the fundus. Representative sections are submitted in eight cassettes:

Cassette A1 – anterior cervix.
Cassette A2 – posterior cervix.
Cassette A3 – anterior lower uterine segment.
Cassette A4 – posterior uterine lower segment.
Cassette A5 – anterior endometrium.
Cassette A6 – posterior endometrium.
Cassettes A7 and A8 – nodules.

Microscopic examination

After gross examination of the tissue, selected tissue (for larger specimens) or biopsy tissue is placed inside a plastic tissue cassette labeled with the case number. This cassette is placed in formalin and goes through a series of dehydration steps in different solutions. My laboratory has computerized processors that change the solutions on a fixed time schedule. Depending on the types of cases seen, a laboratory may have a processing machine dedicated to “rush” cases, with shorter processing time. Because the processing goes along a specific schedule, missing a cutoff time means a case cannot be appropriately processed and has to wait until the next run. Thus, it is important for clinicians to be aware that there are times tissue can be rushed for the same day and other times when this may not be possible. A telephone call to the pathologist discussing the nature of the problem and the reason for the rush is often helpful in these instances. The request for a “rush” on a specimen should be a judicious one.

After the tissue has been processed and is dehydrated, it is removed from the plastic cassette and embedded in paraffin on the outside of the cassette, creating a tissue block. The tissue block is placed on a microtome, a device that allows extremely thin slices to be cut from the block, approximately 4.5 μm. Hence, many slices can be cut from a single block, up to 50–100, depending on the size of the tissue. The microtome produces ribbons of tissue, multiple slices in series, which are floated on a warm water bath, picked up onto glass slides, stained, cover-slipped, and labeled. If duplicate slides are needed for performing special stains such as immunohistochemistry or for outside consultation, they can be *recut* from the block. If a tiny area suggests that there is more of a lesion in the block to be evaluated, *levels* can be cut. Levels differ from recuts, which are the next adjacent section. Levels are cut beyond a "skip area" between the previous slide and the next one, with the aim of identifying a lesion further into the block (**Figures 1.1** and **1.2**).

Laboratories are required to keep slides and tissue blocks for a number of years, which may vary by laboratory location. This is important if future studies or evaluations are needed.

Pathology reports

In addition to patient demographics, the requisition slip should also contain the source of the specimen, the procedure that was performed,

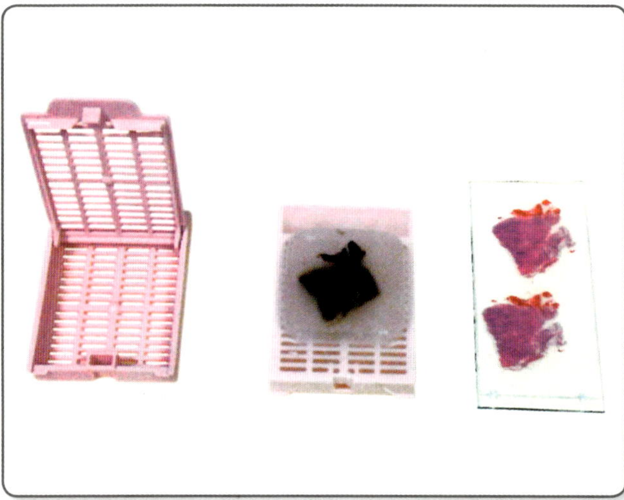

Figure 1.1 Left to right: empty tissue cassette, tissue block, slide prepared from this block.

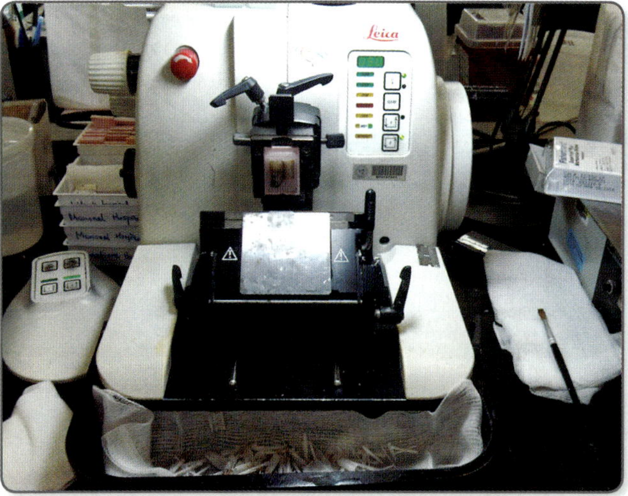

Figure 1.2 Microtome holding block. Note the shaved trimmings in basket.

and any clinical information that is relevant, including any prior hormonal therapy, last menstrual period or menopausal status, pertinent prior surgery, working diagnosis, etc. These will be entered onto the final pathology report, along with the gross description, and final diagnosis. A specific microscopic description of what is seen is included in the report by some laboratories but not by others. Also sometimes included are specific comments by the pathologist, focusing on key diagnostic features or recommendations. This is also often where results of additional testing, such as immunohistochemistry, cytogenetics, or molecular diagnostics are reported.

A question that comes up at times is whether or not to put multiple biopsies in the same jar. This is more relevant to cervical than endometrial biopsies. There is a separate charge for each jar, and a separate diagnosis on the report. It would not be advisable to put an endometrial curettage and an endocervical curettage in the same jar, as separate information will not be possible, and the endocervical component, if scanty, may be overlooked. For hysterectomies with lymph node sampling, laterality or localization of the nodes may be important clinically, and hence separate jars should be used. The bottom line is that if separate diagnoses are needed, separate jars should be used.

Separate final diagnoses are provided in the pathology report for each separate specimen jar. If more than one diagnosis is given for a specimen, they are usually stated in descending order of importance. For cancer resections, (not biopsies), the pathologic TNM classification is often provided as pTNM, to distinguish it from the clinical staging. Terminology for neoplasms usually corresponds to World Health Organization terminology, however it may be variable; this is discussed in the following chapters under specific diagnoses.

If additional stains or levels are obtained, this highlights that a case is more complicated, and perhaps a more difficult differential diagnosis. It will also increase the turnaround time, and may add extra charges to a case. Pathology is a consultative specialty, and cases are often shown to colleagues in the department by the pathologist, and may be sent out for a second or expert opinion in difficult cases. These consultations are generally referenced in the report as well.

A pathology report should be concise, unambiguous, and keyed to current terminology and guidelines for reporting. A clinician should never hesitate to call the pathologist to discuss or explain a report. Such conversations optimize patient care, and are educational on both sides.

Adequacy of specimen

With liberal use of in-office endometrial sampling, the problem of specimens that show only scant superficial endometrial glandular strips on histology has become common[9] (**Figure 1.3**). In the setting of a sample from a postmenopausal woman who has a thin endometrial stripe on ultrasound, this may reflect genuine atrophy; however, it may also reflect insufficient sampling of a nonatrophic uterine cavity.

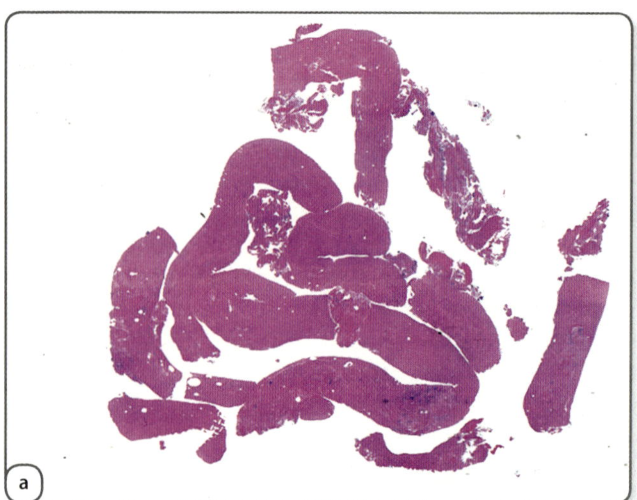

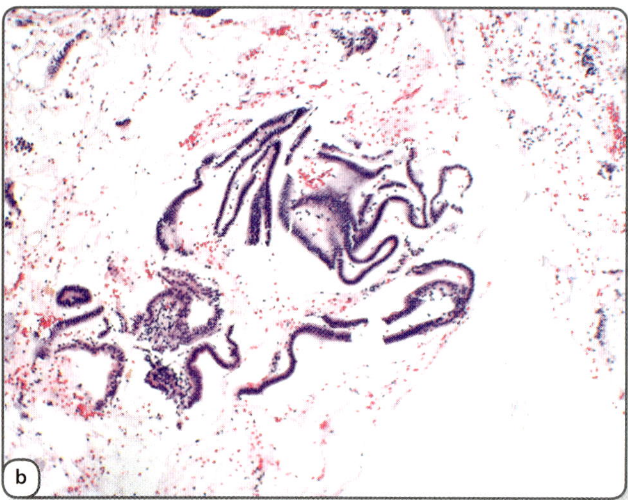

Figure 1.3 Pipelle sampling. (a) Low power view of a Pipelle sample showing what appears to be much tissue, but is actually mostly blood. (b) Strips of benign endometrial glands from pipelle sampling on a recently postmenopausal woman.

The way a report is phrased in these cases is variable. Concern has been raised by some about calling such a specimen "inadequate", as it may be taken as reflecting poor sampling technique, having medicolegal connotations.[10] A statement such as "extremely scanty strips of endometrial glands insufficient for further evaluation" conveys what is present, and allows clinical correlation as to whether sampling was adequate, which is necessary to make this determination. Any atypia should be reported. The presence of mitotic activity, pseudostratification, or tubal metaplasia suggests at least some estrogenic influence (**Figures 1.4–1.7**). While this may not be significant in a recently menopausal woman, it may be of concern in a woman many years remote from the onset of menopause. Clinical judgment is important in these cases, and needs to be correlated with the findings.

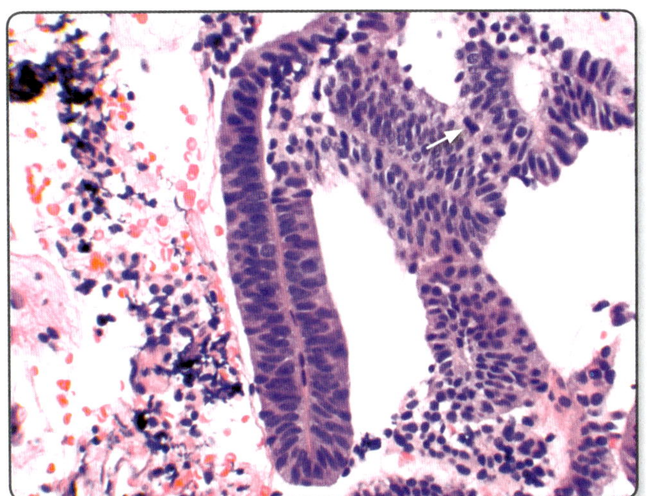

Figure 1.4 Endometrial glandular strips from a biopsy. Presence of pseudostratification and mitosis (arrow) confirm estrogenic effect.

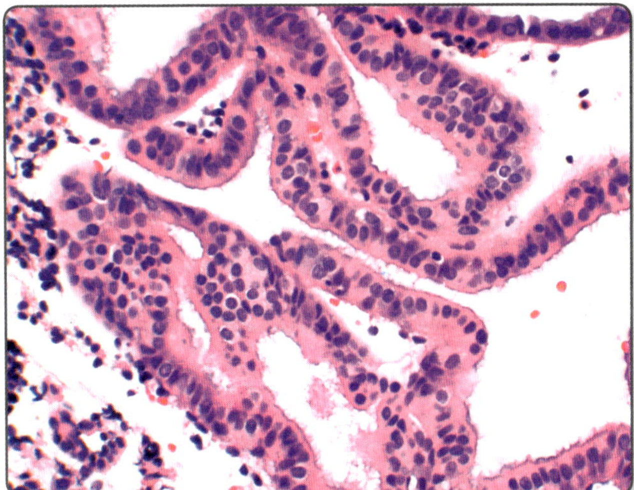

Figure 1.5 Tubal metaplasia on an endometrial biopsy, compatible with prior estrogen effect.

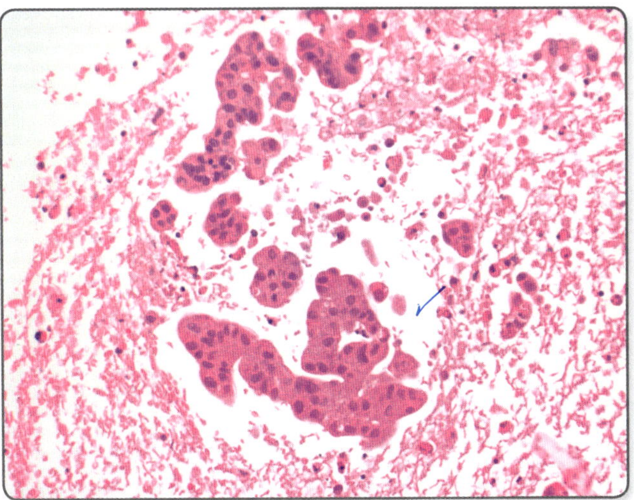

Figure 1.6 Papillary fragments on an endometrial biopsy. This may or may not represent significant pathology, but needs to be reported and evaluated further.

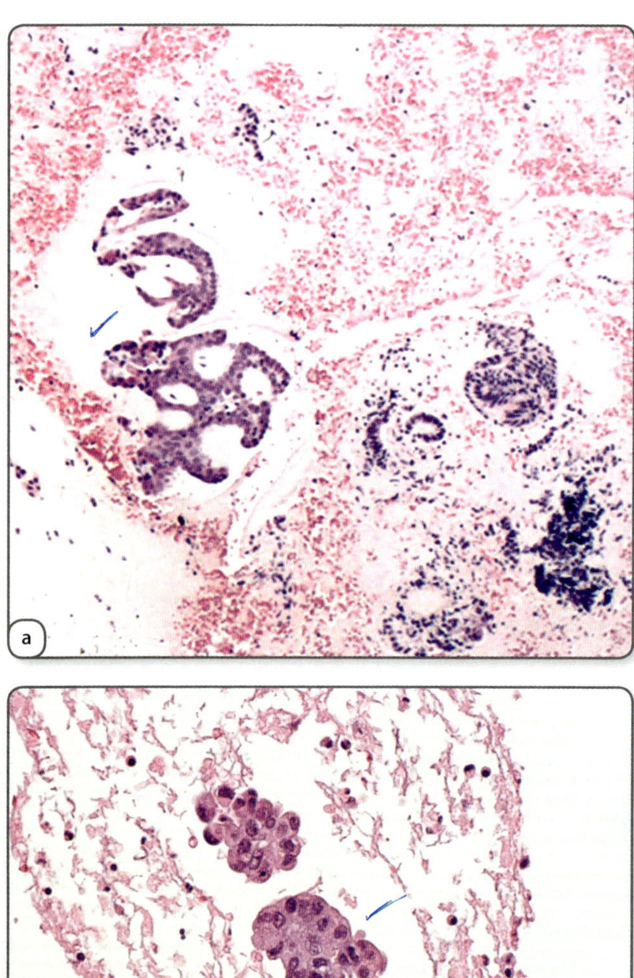

Figure 1.7 Papillary fragments. Follow-up of both these cases revealed endometrial carcinoma.

These strips sometimes assume a pseudopapillary architecture, and this should not be interpreted as a papillary lesion[10].

A variety of conditions may lead to scant tissue, including atrophy, hormonal therapies that suppress the endometrium (such as leuprolide acetate or progestins), prior heavy bleeding, prior curettage, Asherman's syndrome, cervical stenosis, or operator inexperience. Abundant tissue is more likely when there is abundant endometrium present, such as late proliferative endometrium, secretory endometrium, pregnancy-related changes, estrogenic therapy, or hyperplasia/neoplasia.

References

1. Stewart EA, Nowak RA. Leiomyoma-related bleeding: a classic hypothesis updated for the molecular era. Hum Reprod Update 1996;2:295–301.
2. The ESHRE Capri Workshop Group. Endometrial Bleeding. Hum Reprod 2007;13:421–31.
3. Hickey M, Fraser I. Human uterine vascular structures in normal and diseased states. Micros Res Tech 2003;60:377–89.
4. Revel A. Multitasking human endometrium. A review of endometrial biopsy as a diagnostic tool, therapeutic applications, and a source of adult stem cells. Obstet Gynecol Survey 2009;64:249–57.
5. Huang GS, Gebb JS, Einstein MH, Shahabi S, Novetsky A, Goldberg GL. Accuracy of preoperative endometrial sampling for detection of high-grade endometrial tumors. AJOG 2007;196:243.e1–5.
6. Rodriguez GC, Yaqub N, King ME. A comparison of the Pipelle device and the Vabra aspirator as measured by endometrial denudation in hysterectomy specimens: the Pipelle device samples significantly less of the endometrial surface than the Vabra aspirator. Am J Obstet Gynecol 1993;168:55–59.
7. Dijkhuizen FP, Mol BW, Brolmann HA, Heintz AP. The accuracy of endometrial sampling in the diagnosis of patients with endometrial carcinoma and hyperplasia. Cancer 2000;89:1765–72.
8. Williams ARW, Brechin S, Porter AJL, Warner P, Critchley HOD. Factors affecting adequacy of Pipelle and Tao Brush endometrial sampling. BJOG 2008;115:1028–36.
9. McCluggage WG. My approach to the interpretation of endometrial biopsies. J Clin Pathol 2006;59:801–12.
10. McCluggage WG. Miscellaneous disorders involving the endometrium. Semin Diagn Pathol 2010;27:287–310.

2 The normal endometrial cycle

In 1950, Noyes, Hertig and Rock published their sentinel paper on dating the endometrium.[1] They correlated the morphology with clinical cycles, and developed histologic criteria for endometrial dating that are still used today, although less frequently.

Women undergoing infertility evaluations used to have endometrial biopsies routinely to document that ovulation had occurred and that the luteal phase was of appropriate duration and quality. In order to diagnose a luteal phase defect, a lag of at least 2 days between the biopsy and the clinical menstrual date on two separate samplings is needed.[2] However, not all authors are convinced of the association of a lag with clinical fertility issues,[3] and there is much interobserver variability in reading these biopsies.[2,4] Much of the hormonal information can now be determined by serological testing of hormonal levels rather than endometrial biopsy.

With these caveats in mind, a brief description of endometrial dating follows. Although endometrial dating has customarily been based on an idealized 28-day cycle with ovulation occurring at 14 days, many normal women do not have a 28-day cycle. It had been thought that this indicated variations in the length of the preovulatory phase of the cycle, with the postovulatory period a fixed 14 days, but it is now known that the latter may vary as well.[5]

Menstrual/early proliferative endometrium (day 1–5)

The complex hormonal interactions of the feedback loop between the ovaries, pituitary and hypothalamus have been well documented. The biological purpose of the menstrual cycle is to support a gestation. If pregnancy does not occur, a new cycle starts, resulting in subsequent ovulation.

The drop in estrogen and progesterone production by the regressing corpus luteum of the prior cycle allows negative feedback to the central nervous system to be removed, resulting in increasing FSH (follicle stimulating hormone), and follicular maturation. This reduction in estrogen and progesterone also leads to sloughing of the secretory endometrium (menses). Rising estrogen production by recruited follicles of the new cycle allows regeneration and development of proliferative endometrium again. Because only the upper endometrium sloughs, the remaining basal endometrium is available to give rise to the endometrial lining of each subsequent cycle.

The menstrual phase is generally considered to be the first 5 days of the cycle, although this is variable from woman to woman. It is also the early proliferative phase, and so a mixture of changes associated with menses and with the early proliferative endometrium is seen. Menstrual endometrium is characterized by an influx of inflammatory cells into the endometrium, thrombi in stromal vessels, apoptosis, and gland-stromal dissociation (**Figures 2.1–2.6**). The presence of inflammatory cells should not be construed as endometritis, which will be discussed further in the next chapter. The dissociation of the glands from the stroma leads to stromal aggregates, which appear darker, giving

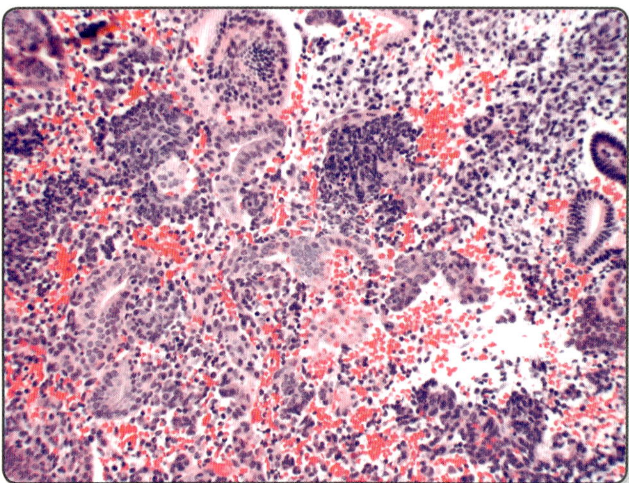

Figure 2.1 Menstrual endometrium. Note complete fragmentation and separation of glands and stroma.

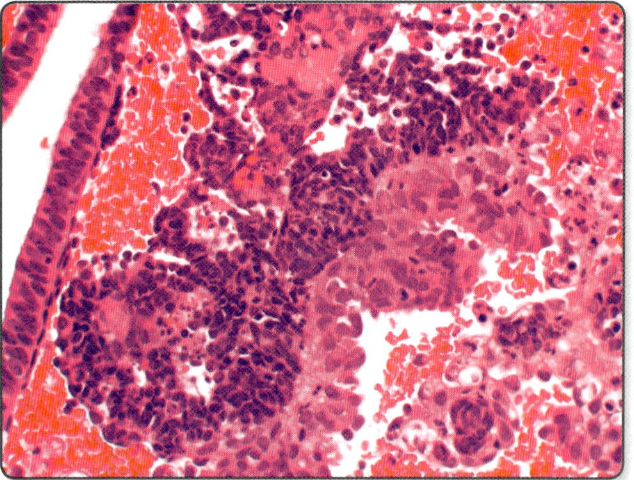

Figure 2.2 Menstrual endometrium. Often the glandular epithelium appears lighter, and the stroma darker. The arrowhead points to the nuclear dust of apoptosis.

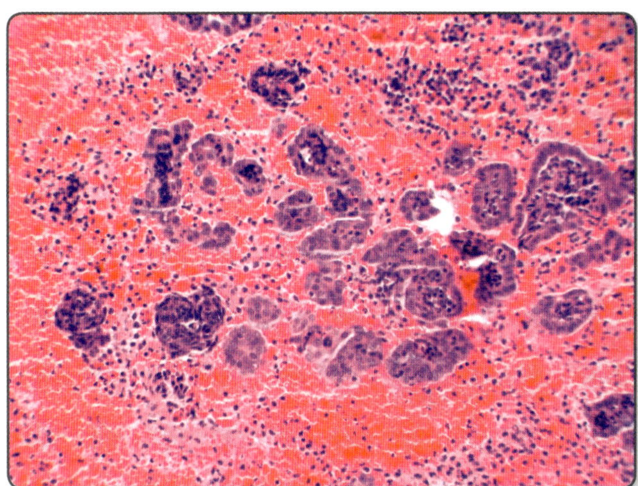

Figure 2.3 Menstrual endometrium. Fragmentation leads to clusters of stromal aggregates ("blue balls"). Some of these are surrounded by glandular epithelium. This structure is termed "exodus" if seen on a Pap smear.

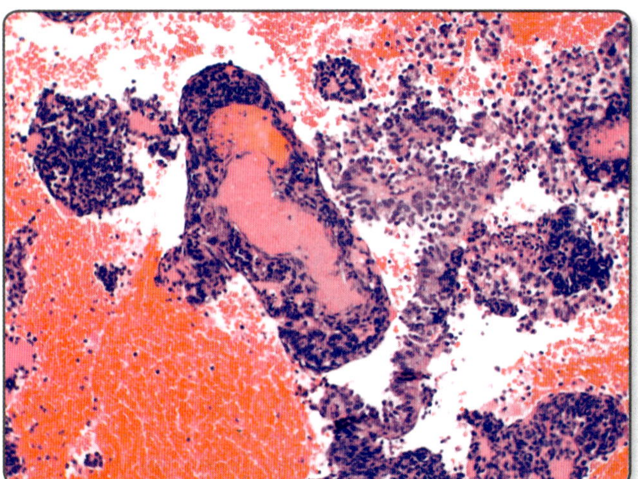

Figure 2.4 Menstrual endometrium with thrombosis of stromal vessels.

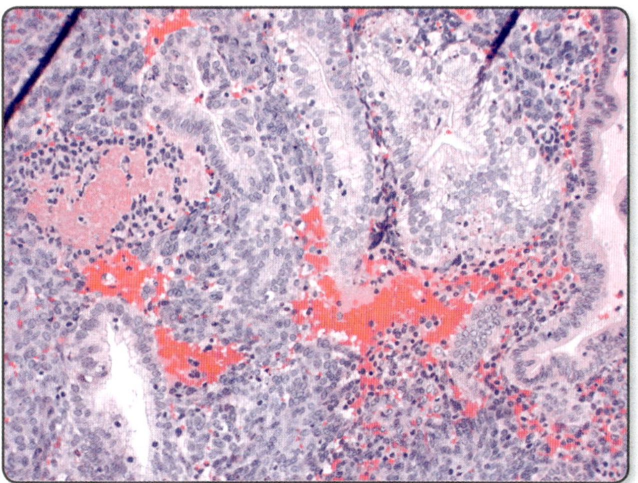

Figure 2.5 Menstrual endometrium. Artifactual vacuolization can be seen, and should not be interpreted as secretory change in the glands.

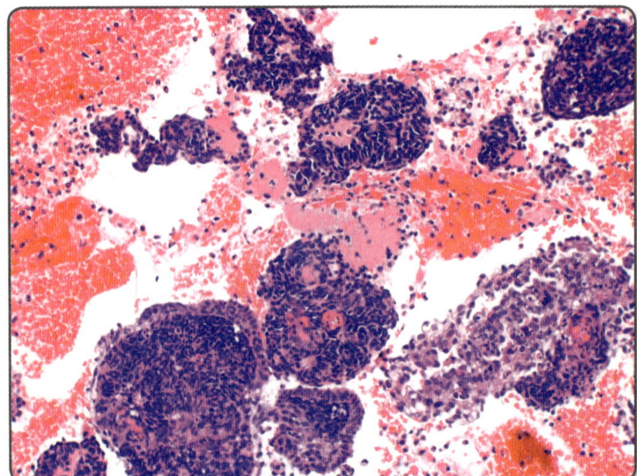

Figure 2.6 Menstrual endometrium showing several stromal "blue balls". In the left lower corner, a stromal aggregate surrounded by glandular epithelium ("exodus") is seen.

rise to the descriptive term "blue balls". The disruption of the glands may cause them to appear closer together than they were previously. In the presence of endometrial breakdown, it may not be possible to determine whether or not ovulation has occurred, in which case the term "shedding endometrium" may be more appropriate, as clinicians may interpret "menstrual endometrium' to mean that ovulation has occurred. In the presence of marked endometrial breakdown, whether ovulatory menstrual, or due to anovulatory causes (see Chapter 5), the close apposition of the glands due to loss of the "scaffolding", should not be construed as hyperplasia.

The histologic features of endometrial breakdown described above may overlap and persist into the early proliferative phase. Early proliferative endometrium is composed of straight, relatively uncoiled glands, and configuration may best be appreciated on a hysterectomy specimen. On biopsy or curettage, the glands are most often seen in cross section, and look like "little blue donuts", small circular glands. The epithelium is pseudostratified. This means that while nuclei may be seen at various levels of the epithelium, all epithelial cells are in contact with the basement membrane of the gland, hence not truly stratified. Mitotic activity may be seen in the glands and stroma over the proliferative period, increasing along the cycle (**Figures 2.7–2.9**).

Mid- to late proliferative endometrium (days 6–14)

From the mid- to late proliferative period, there is increased coiling of glands, and increased mitotic activity in both glands and stroma (**Figures 2.10–2.12 a** and **b**). There may be stromal edema during the midproliferative phase, however this is not always seen. In reality, dating of proliferative endometrium is not utilized clinically, and so a diagnosis of proliferative endometrium is sufficient.

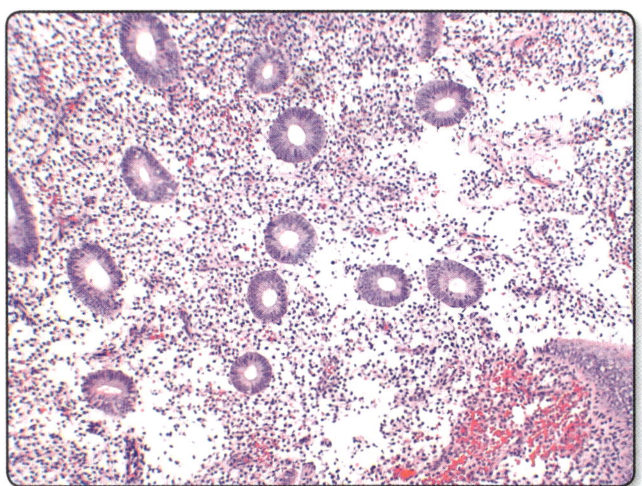

Figure 2.7 Early proliferative endometrium. In cross section, the glands look like "little blue donuts".

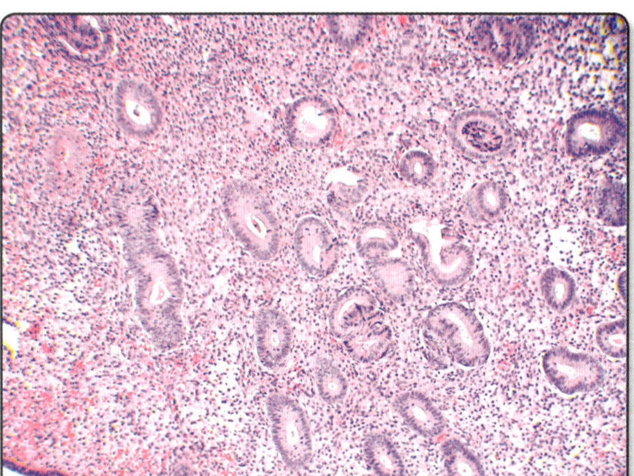

Figure 2.8 Early proliferative endometrium. Longitudinal sections of the glands show relatively uncoiled glands

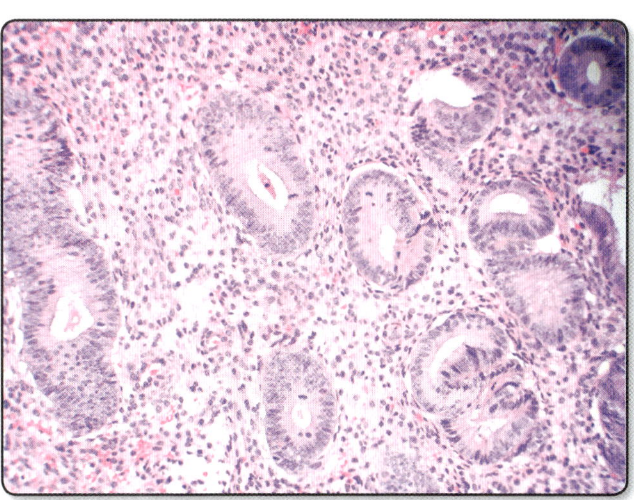

Figure 2.9 Early proliferative endometrium. Higher power shows pseudostratification of the glandular epithelium. Several mitotic figures are seen in the glands.

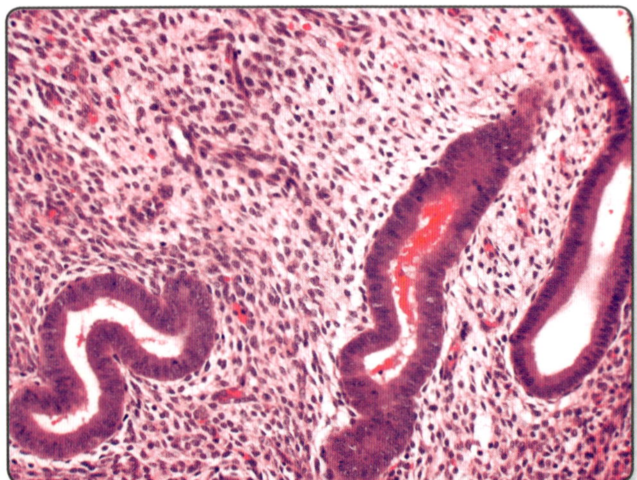

Figure 2.10 Midproliferative endometrium, showing beginning coiling of glands, and mild stromal edema.

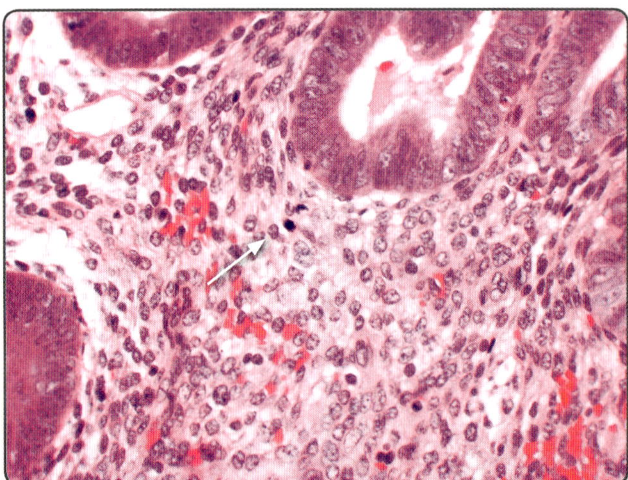

Figure 2.11 Midproliferative endometrium. Stromal mitotic figures (arrow) are easily seen.

There are a few possible pitfalls in evaluating this endometrium. The nuclei have coarse chromatin, however gland and nuclear arrangements are orderly, hence this should not be interpreted as neoplastic. The spindled stroma may be misinterpreted as predecidua, however the mitotic activity militates against a secretory endometrium.[2] Likewise, scattered intraluminal material in the glands, or subnuclear vacuoles are not proof positive of ovulation, and may be estrogen effect alone. The increased tortuosity of the glands in late proliferative endometrium may appear as crowded glands on cross section, and should not be interpreted as hyperplasia. In processing, intussusception or telescoping of the glands may occur, and this too should not be interpreted as hyperplasia[2] (**Figure 2.12c**).

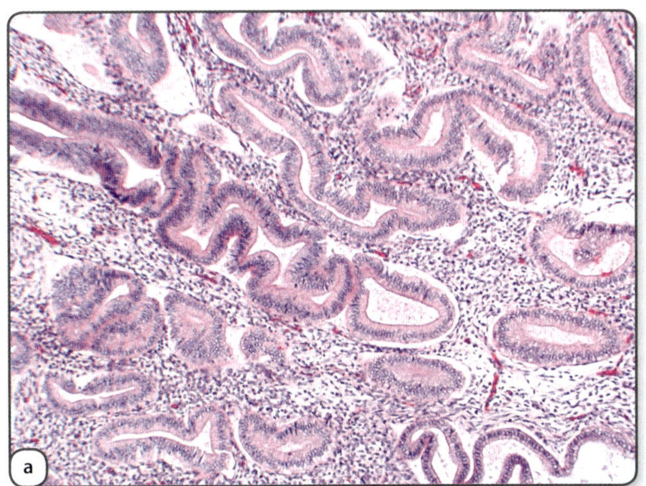

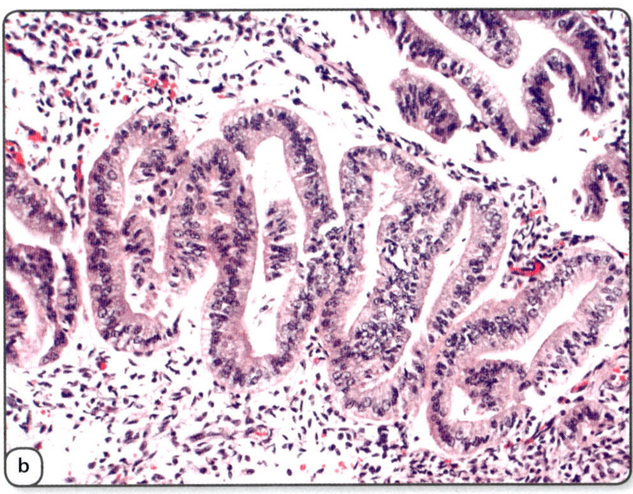

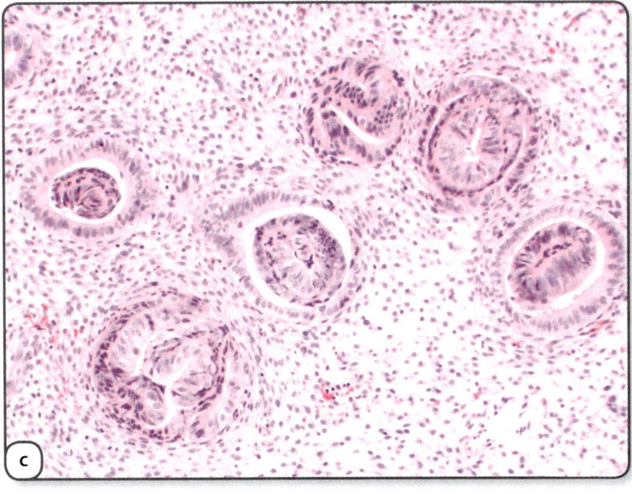

Figure 2.12 Late proliferative endometrium, showing extensive coiling of glands (a). This can appear as numerous glands in cross section, and should not be interpreted as glandular crowding or hyperplasia (b). Telescoping artifact does not represent hyperplasia (c).

Interval endometrium (day 15–16, postovulatory day (POD) 2–3)

Interval endometrium has features of both proliferative and secretory endometrium. Subnuclear vacuoles are present, although in less than 50% of the glands. Mitoses persist, only to disappear later in the secretory phase. The glands overall still have a proliferative architecture. However, the features of interval endometrium can be seen whether or not ovulation has occurred, and hence the pathologist cannot confirm that ovulation has occurred on the basis of this morphology (**Figure 2.13**)

Secretory endometrium (day 17–28, POD 4–14)

The portion of the menstrual cycle most amenable to morphologic endometrial dating is from day 17–28 (**Table 2.1**). Day 17 is one of the most recognizable days, with uniform subnuclear vacuoles under the epithelial nuclei, which are closer to the gland lumens. This gives a "piano key" appearance (**Figure 2.14**). Rare mitoses may still be seen. The epithelium is no longer pseudostratified in appearance but appears as a single layer.

The next few days of the cycle are focused on the glands, with movement of the vacuoles towards the gland lumens, and secretion into the glands. Day 18 is characterized by vacuoles both above and below gland nuclei (**Figure 2.15**). By day 19, vacuoles are above gland nuclei. Peak secretion is seen on day 20. The apical portions of the glands may have "snouts". The rest of the secretory phase occurs in the stroma, as the glands become exhausted, and take on a sawtooth appearance. By day 21, there is beginning stromal edema. The features seen on days 19–21 may overlap, and make it difficult to assign an exact day to 'the tissue (**Figure 2.16**). Peak stromal edema is seen on day 22 (**Figure 2.17**). By day 23, the glands show sawtooth infoldings consistent with secretory exhaustion, and the

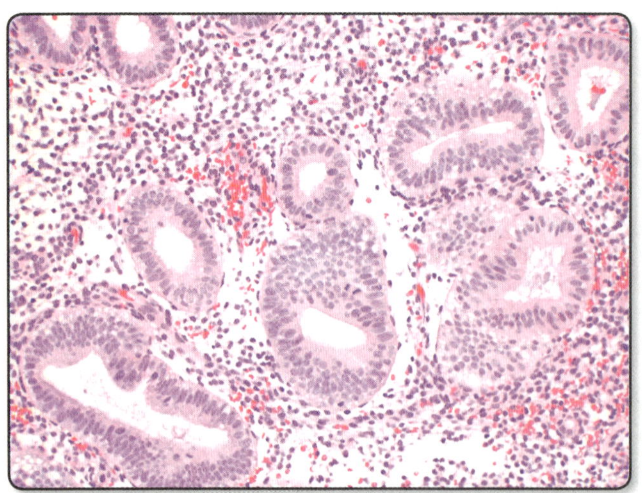

Figure 2.13 Interval endometrium. Subnuclear vacuoles are seen, however the glands are still of proliferative pseudostratified architecture, and a mitotic figure is seen.

Dating the endometrium	
Date	**Features**
Menses/day 28 (POD 14)	Breakdown
Early proliferative	Residual breakdown. Straight tubular glands ("little blue donuts"), mitoses in glands/stroma
Midproliferative	Increasing gland tortuosity, mitoses in glands/stroma, possibly stroma more edematous
Late Proliferative	Greater gland tortuosity, stroma no longer edematous. Mitoses in glands/stroma
Interval day 16 (POD 2)	Overall proliferative pattern, with subnuclear vacuoles in about 50% of glands
Day 17 (POD 3)	Piano-key subnuclear vacuoles. Mitoses rare after this.
Day 18 (POD 4)	Vacuoles both above and below gland nuclei
Day 19 (POD 5)	Vacuoles above gland nuclei
Day 20 (POD 6)	Peak secretion
Day 21 (POD 7)	Beginning stromal edema
Day 22 (POD 8)	Peak stromal edema
Day 23 (POD 9)	Glands with secretory exhaustion, spiral arterioles prominent
Day 24 (POD 10)	Glands with secretory exhaustion, spiral arterioles with predecidual cuffing
Day 25 (POD 11)	Glands with secretory exhaustion, spiral arterioles with predecidual cuffing, predecidua under surface epithelium
Day 26 (POD 12)	Glands with secretory exhaustion, expanding predecidua
Day 27 (POD 13)	Glands with secretory exhaustion, entire stroma predecidualized. Influx of inflammatory cells

POD, postovulatory day.

Table 2.1 Dating the endometrium

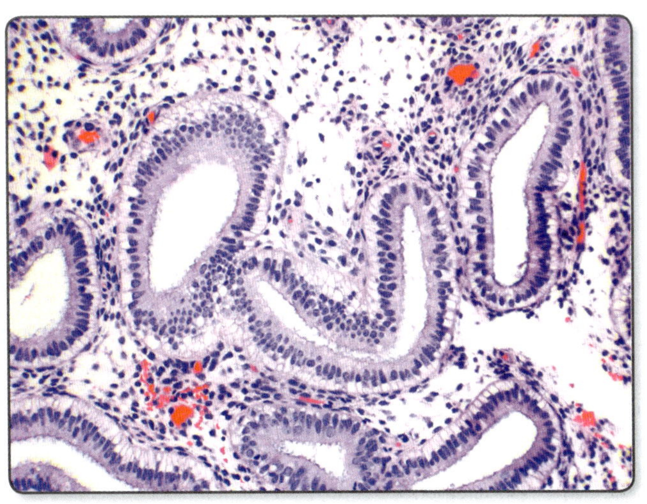

Figure 2.14 17-day secretory endometrium showing uniform subnuclear vacuoles. The glandular epithelium appears as a single layer, and mitoses are not evident.

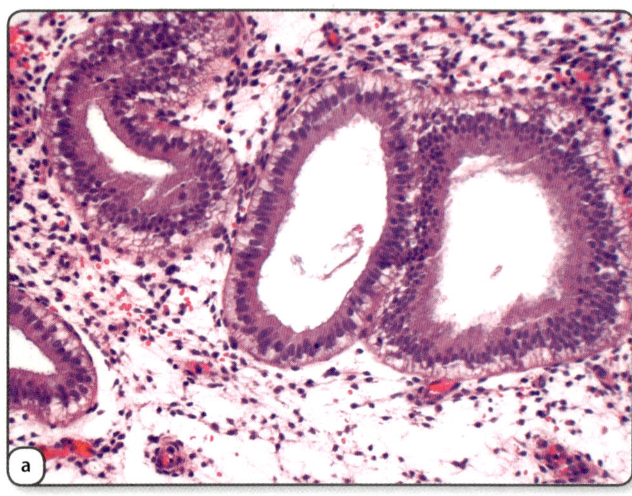

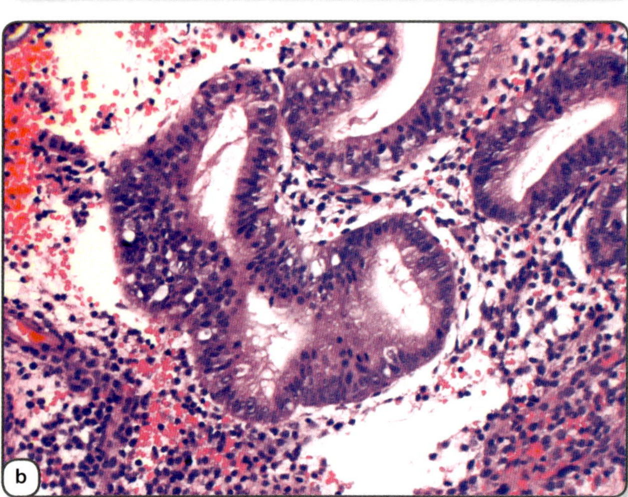

Figure 2.15 18-day secretory endometrium showing vacuoles both above and below the nuclei (a). Rare mitoses may still be seen (b).

spiral arterioles are seen prominently in the stroma. In cross section, these spiraling vessels are seen as multiple circular structures in a cluster (**Figure 2.18**). Day 24 shows glands with more secretory exhaustion, and the spiral arterioles have a predecidual cuffing (**Figure 2.19**). The predecidua expands for the rest of the cycle. In addition to marked glandular secretory exhaustion and spiral arterioles with predecidual cuffing, on day 25, predecidua is also under the surface epithelium (**Figure 2.20**). Expanding predecidua is seen on day 26, until on day 27 the entire stroma is predecidualized (**Figure 2.21**). There is the beginning of influx of inflammatory cells on day 27, peaking on the beginning of menses, day 28 (**Figure 2.22**), when gland-stromal dissociation begins. Neutrophils and lymphocytes may be seen in the stroma, however plasma cells are not expected and, if present, indicate chronic endometritis. The inflammatory cells seen just prior and during menses should not be interpreted as acute or chronic endometritis (see Chapter 4).

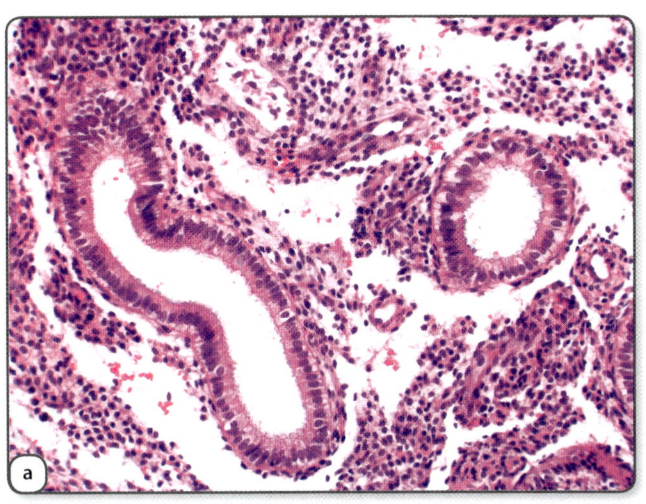

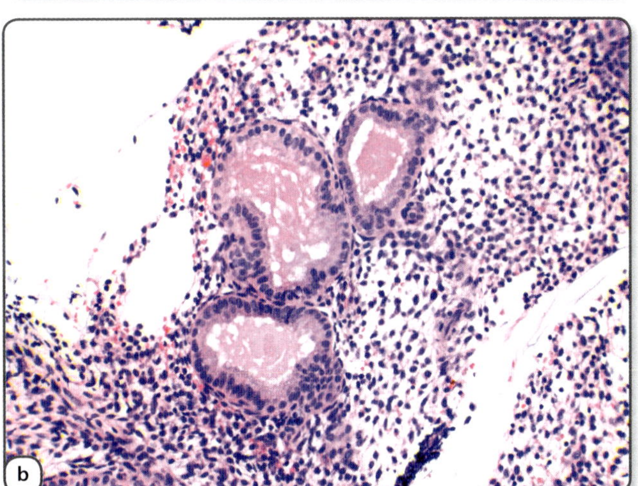

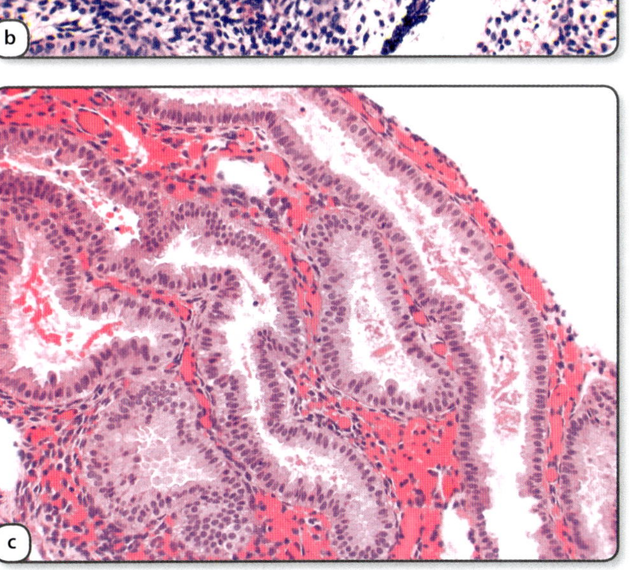

Figure 2.16 19- to 21-day secretory endometrium. The features of endometrium between these days are often too indistinct to assign a single date. The vacuoles have entirely migrated to the luminal surface by day 19 (a), and peak secretion is seen at day 20 (b). Beginning stromal edema occurs on day 21. Notice the apocrine snouts on the apical surface of the glandular epithelium (c).

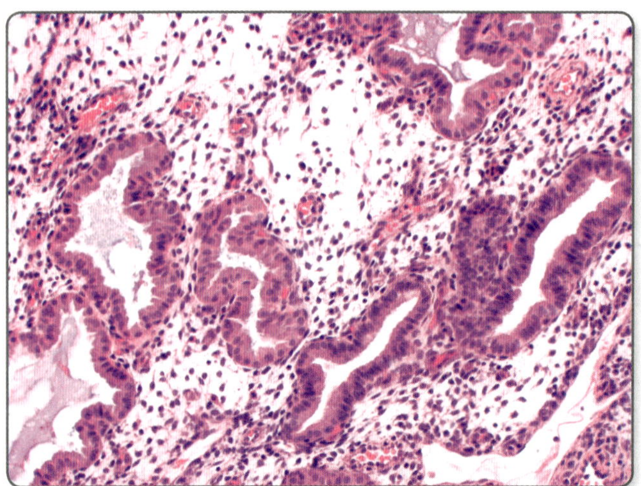

Figure 2.17 22-day secretory endometrium with stromal edema.

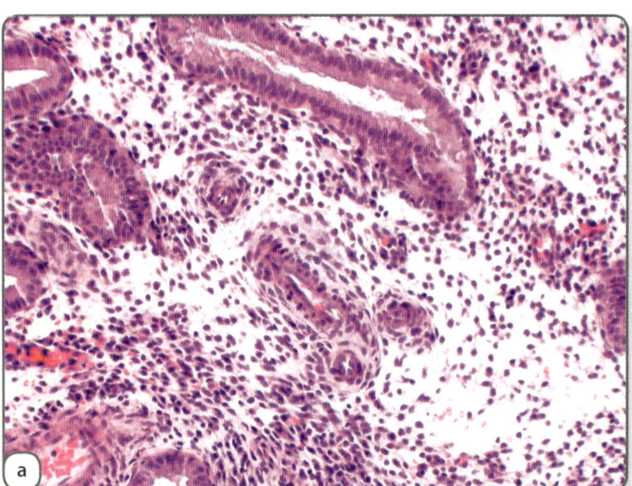

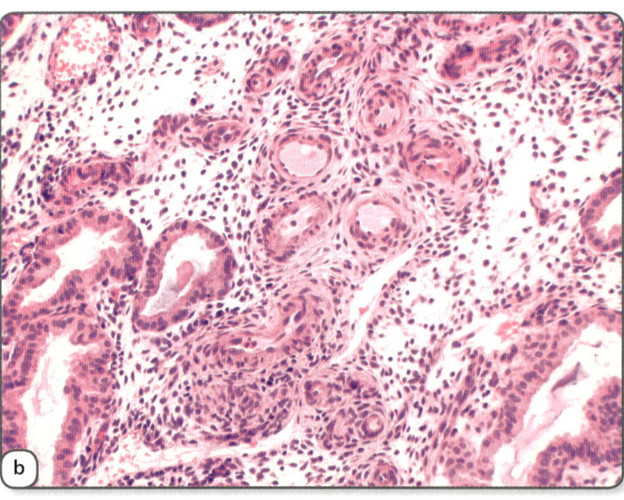

Figure 2.18 23-day secretory endometrium showing prominent spiral arterioles (a), which start to develop a predecidual cuff (b).

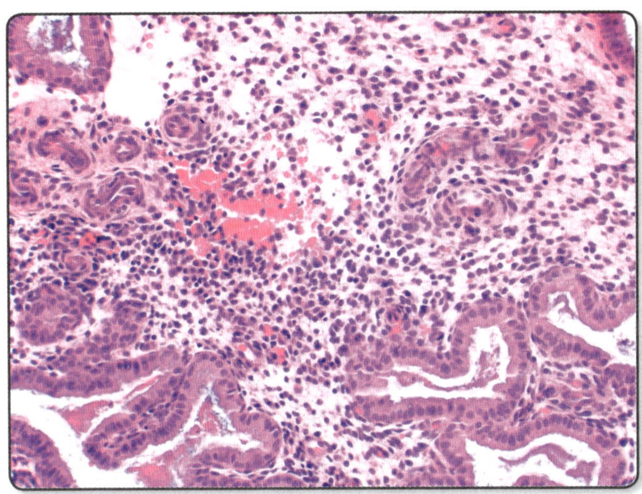

Figure 2.19 24-day secretory endometrium. The predecidual cuff around the spiral arterioles is more expanded than day 23.

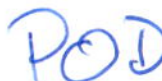

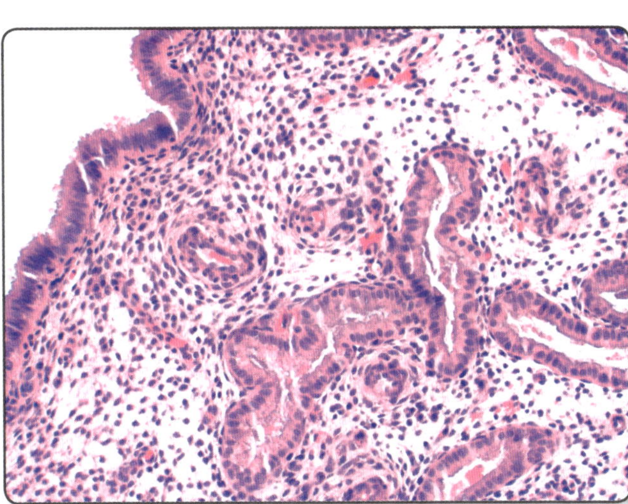

Figure 2.20 25-day secretory endometrium. In addition to expanded periarteriolar predecidua, the predecidual change is seen under the surface endometrium. This is best appreciated at low power, and intact fragments with surface epithelium are needed to see this feature.

Atrophic endometrium

In menopausal women the lack of hormonal stimulation leads to endometrial atrophy, with nonsecretory glands that have a flattened epithelium and are devoid of mitotic activity (**Figure 2.23**). The glands may become cystic, and it is the flattened nonproliferating nature of the epithelium that distinguishes cystic atrophy from simple hyperplasia.

Luteal phase defects

A luteal phase defect is a clinical rather than pathological diagnosis, marked by a lag of more than 2 days in the development of the secretory endometrium, on biopsies on two separate occasions. Hence, the dates of the subsequent menstrual period must be known to be able to make this determination, as there can also be delayed ovulation.

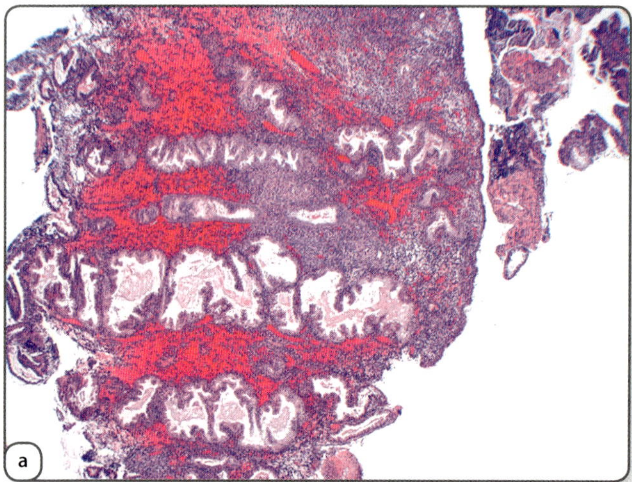

Figure 2.21 27-day secretory endometrium, showing predecidualization of the entire stroma and secretorily exhausted glands (a, b).

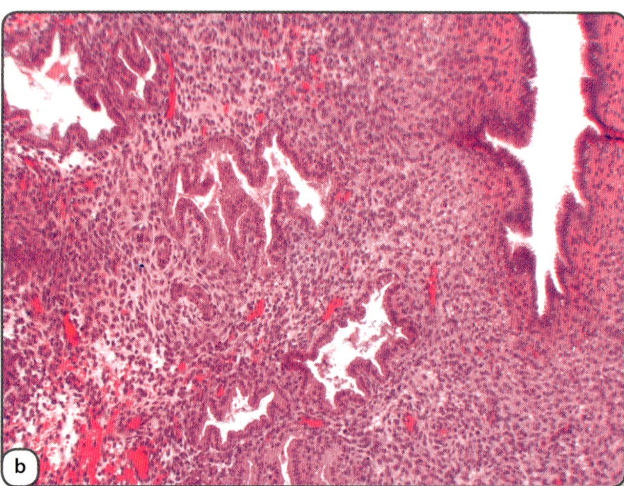

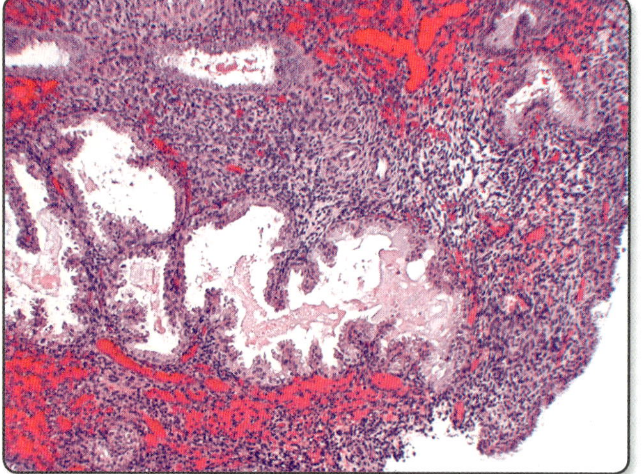

Figure 2.22 Secretory day 28, early hemorrhage on day 28. Not shown are inflammatory cells and areas of gland stromal dissociation as menses ensues.

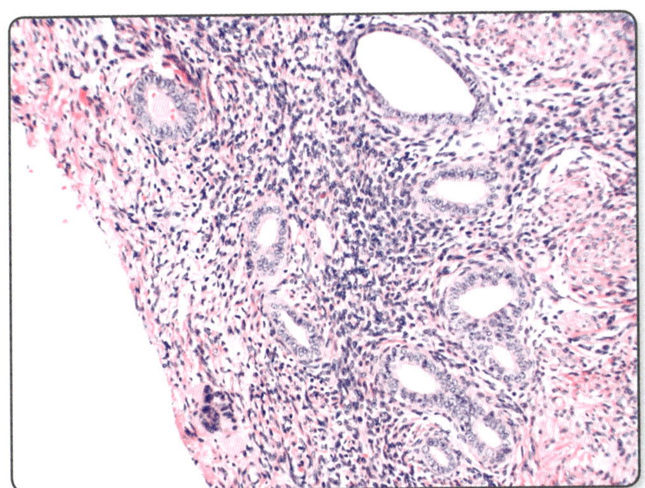

Figure 2.23 Atrophic endometrium. Glands are nonsecretory, and the epithelium is flat, without pseudostratification or mitoses.

There are several patterns of abnormally developed secretory endometrium that may be seen, these are thought to relate to abnormalities of the function of the corpus luteum.[6] Dyssynchronously developed endometrium, where the dating of the glands lags behind the stroma, is most often seen after induction of ovulation, but it can be occur spontaneously. The glands usually have a day 17–18 configuration, while the more advanced stroma is often in the range of day 23–24 (**Figure 2.24**).

Two mixed patterns may be seen: irregular shedding (**Figure 2.25**) and irregular ripening (**Figure 2.26**). These occur at different times of the cycle. Irregular shedding is the persistence of secretory changes into the next proliferative phase, due to continued luteal function (lack of regression of the corpus luteum). Hence, the biopsy must be taken no earlier than cycle day 5 to make the diagnosis.

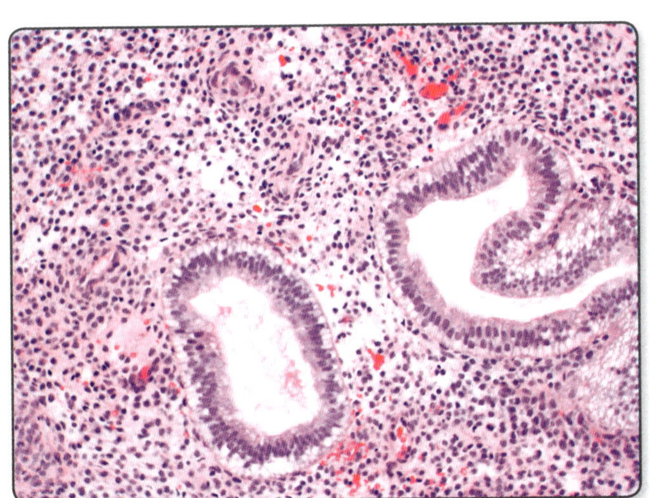

Figure 2.24 Irregularly developed secretory endometrium, with glandular features of day 17, and stromal features of day 23–24.

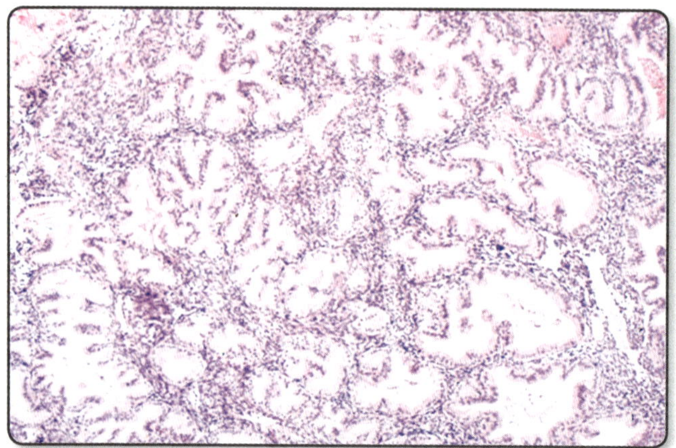

Figure 2.25 Irregular shedding. There is exaggerated secretory exhaustion in this biopsy from the proliferative phase.

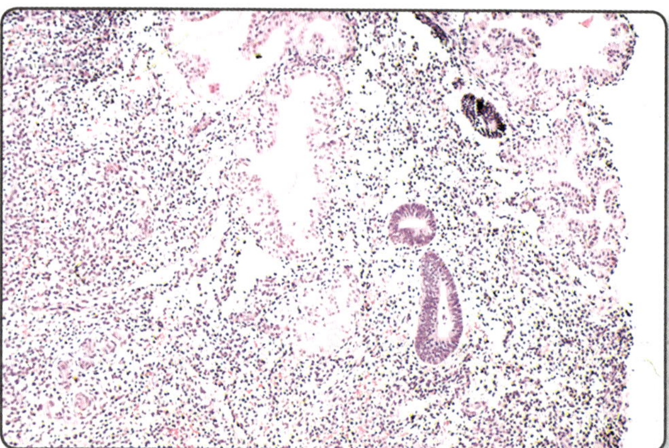

Figure 2.26 Irregular ripening. A few proliferative glands are seen persisting in a late secretory endometrium.

Mixed endometrium is seen, with exaggerated secretorily exhausted glands admixed with proliferative changes. Irregular ripening may be seen in the secretory phase, and is the presence of nonsecretory glands within the stroma of a secretory endometrium, possibly due to a local receptor defect.

References

1. Noyes FW, Hertig AT, Rock J. Dating the endometrial biopsy. Fertil Steril 1950;1:3–25.
2. Crum CP, Hornstein MD, Nucci MR, Mutter GL. Hertig and beyond: a systematic and practical approach to the endometrial biopsy. Adv Anat Pathol 2003;10:301–18.
3. Bukulmez O, Arici A Luteal phase defect: myth or reality. Obstet Gynecol Clin North Am 2004;31:727–44.
4. Duggan MA, Brashert P, Ostor A, Scurry J, Billson V, Kneafsey P, Difrancesco L. The accuracy and interobserver reproducibility of endometrial dating. Pathol 2001; 33:292–97.
5. Fehring RJ, Schneider M, Raviele K. Variability in the phases of the menstrual cycle. J Obstet Gynecol Neonatal Nurs 2006 35:376–84.
6. Deligdisch L. Hormonal pathology of the endometrium. Mod Pathol 2000;13:285–94.

3 Pregnancy-related findings in normal and abnormal pregnancies

Abnormal uterine bleeding in the reproductive age group always raises the possibility of a pregnancy-related condition. This chapter reviews the most commonly encountered pathology specimens.

First trimester intrauterine products of conception

Viable first trimester uterine contents

Generally, the diagnosis of viable first trimester products of conception is not difficult. First trimester villi have a two-cell layer of inner cytotrophoblast and outer syncytiotrophoblast (**Figure 3.1**). Villous trophoblast proliferation is prominent in the first trimester, but usually is focused at one end of the villi, in the direction of implantation, the so-called "polar-capping" (**Figure 3.2**). Capillaries may be seen in the villous stroma, along with Hofbauer cells. Nucleated red blood cells in fetal capillaries are most prominent between 8 and 12 weeks of gestational age. This evidence of a fetal circulation can be used

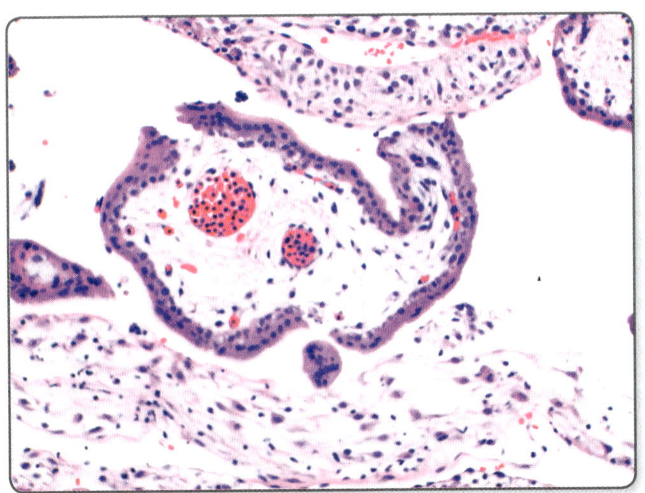

Figure 3.1 First trimester villus showing inner cytotrophoblast layer, outer syncytiotrophoblast layer, and abundant nucleated red blood cells in fetal vessels in the villus.

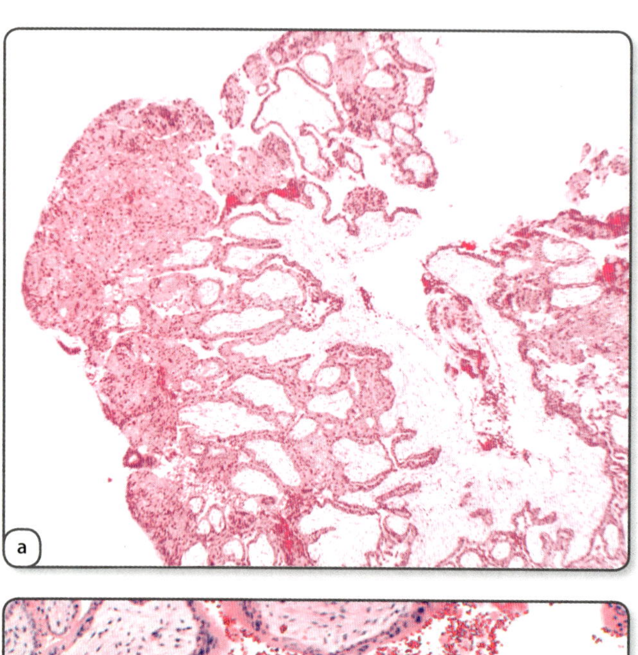

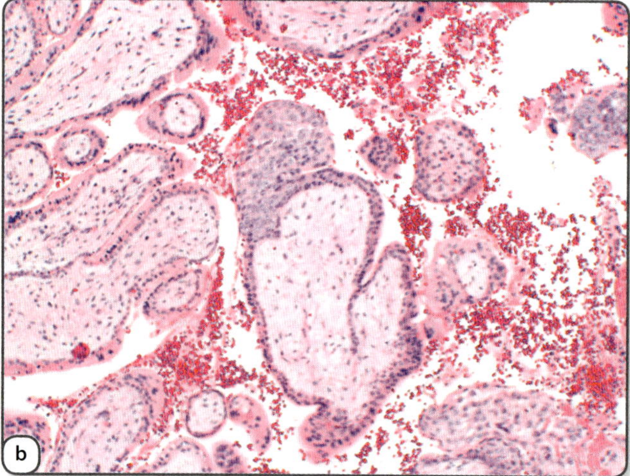

Figure 3.2 Polar-capping. In normal first trimester villi, the trophoblast proliferation is aimed towards the implantation site.

as one of the findings supporting a partial over a complete mole if molar pregnancy is of concern (see p. 41). By the second trimester, the cytotrophoblast layer is less prominent, and hard to identify on routine histology. Third trimester villi are much smaller due to branching, with villous capillaries migrating out towards the edge of the villi, forming vasculosyncytial membranes, which allow for maximum exchange between mother and fetus. Fetal parts are usually easily recognized by 9 weeks in elective termination specimens, although they may be seen before.

The endometrium in the first trimester of pregnancy shows features similar to those seen on day 27 (late secretory), with more prominence of the decidualization, and secretory glandular changes. In areas where the stroma is predominant, this tissue is usually referred to as decidua (as opposed to predecidua before pregnancy) (**Figure 3.3**). In areas where glands are more prominent, the endometrial lining is termed hypersecretory endometrium or gestational endometrium (**Figure 3.4**); however, it is the same tissue as the decidua, the uterine lining.

Arias-Stella reaction

The glands of gestational endometrium may show a hobnail pattern with prominent nuclear atypia, the "Arias-Stella" reaction (**Figure 3.5**), which is due to the influence of hormones. This should not be confused with the tubulopapillary pattern of clear cell adenocarcinoma.

In a recent paper revisiting the entity he described over 40 years ago, Dr Arias-Stella has reviewed the history of his description of the finding.[1] It can be associated with viable or nonviable intrauterine or

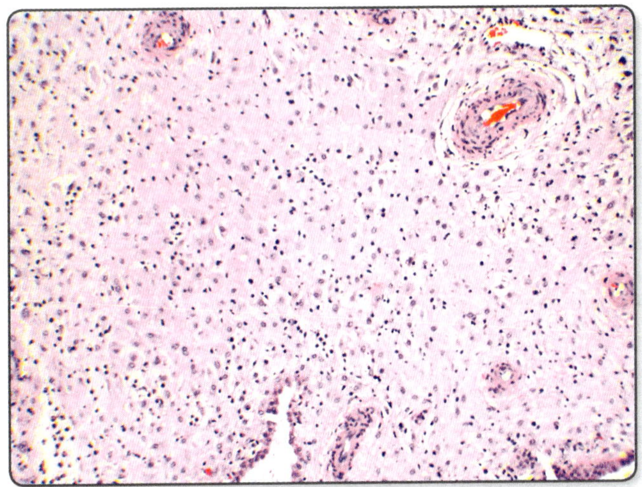

Figure 3.3 Decidua. The decidual changes are more prominent than during the menstrual cycle, with stromal cells showing abundant eosinophilic cytoplasm, and cells having well-defined borders.

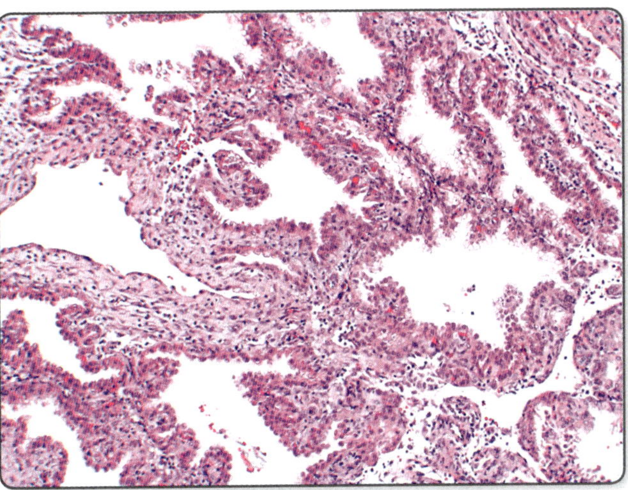

Figure 3.4 Hypersecretory endometrium. Gestational endometrium shows hypersecretory glands, in a decidualized stroma.

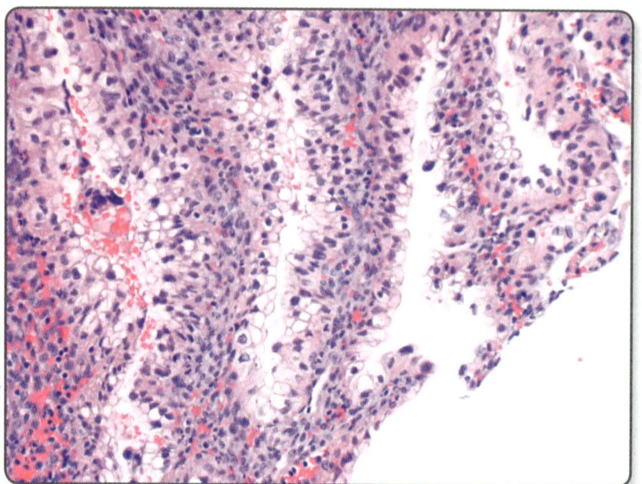

Figure 3.5 Arias-Stella change. Note the hobnailed glandular cells, with atypical nuclei.

ectopic pregnancies, or gestational trophoblastic disease. Nevertheless, it should not be assumed that a gestation is ectopic just because the Arias-Stella reaction is present. Interpretation of the Arias-Stella reaction may become problematic if seen in an older patient who is less likely to raise the clinical impression of pregnancy, or if it is seen as an aftermath of a pregnancy that is no longer ongoing, and may also be potentially be confused with clear cell adenocarcinoma, serous carcinoma or its putative early lesion endometrial intraepithelial carcinoma (EIC). In one study, immunohistochemical staining with Ki-67, a marker of proliferation, and p53 was useful in distinguishing the Arias-Stella reaction from these high-grade carcinomas, which stain significantly more for Ki-67 and p53 than Arias-Stella reaction does.[2]

Missed abortions

A *missed abortion* is the loss of viability of a pregnancy without (or prior to) passage of the products of conception. A fetus may or may not be identifiable, and may have been reabsorbed or never present ("blighted ovum"). After spontaneous passage of the products of conception, a *spontaneous abortion*, either incomplete or complete, is diagnosed. Many of these pregnancy losses are due to chromosomal abnormalities, particularly aneuploidy.[3] Histologically, two general categories of features may be noted in clinically missed abortion specimens. One is various degenerative findings. The other is features that may indicate chromosomal abnormalities or gestational trophoblastic neoplasia.

Degenerative changes of villi include loss of fetal vessels, with progressive fibrosis (**Figure 3.6**). Villous edema (**Figure 3.7**) may raise the question of hydatidiform mole, however the lack of trophoblast proliferation rules out that diagnosis. Avascularity of the villi (**Figure 3.8**) may reflect a missed abortion, but villi examined before a well developed circulatory system is established will also lack vessels and therefore clinical correlation of dates is important. The decidua

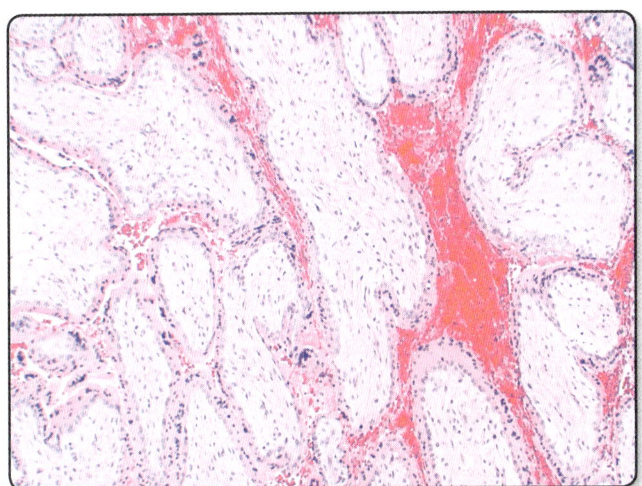

Figure 3.6 Villous fibrosis. Villi have become avascular, with fibrosis of the stroma in a missed abortion.

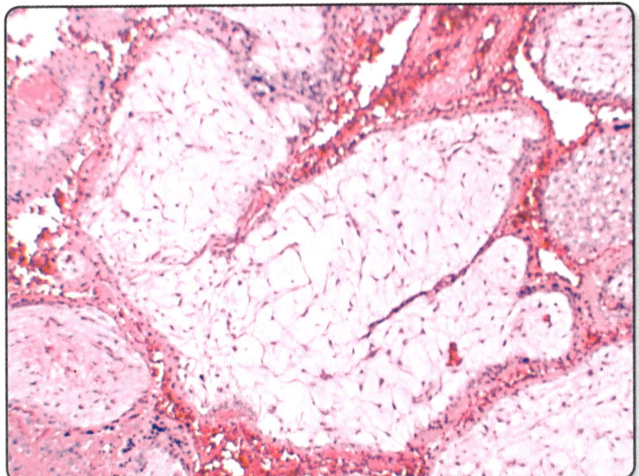

Figure 3.7 Villous edema, in the absence of trophoblast proliferation, is common in missed abortions.

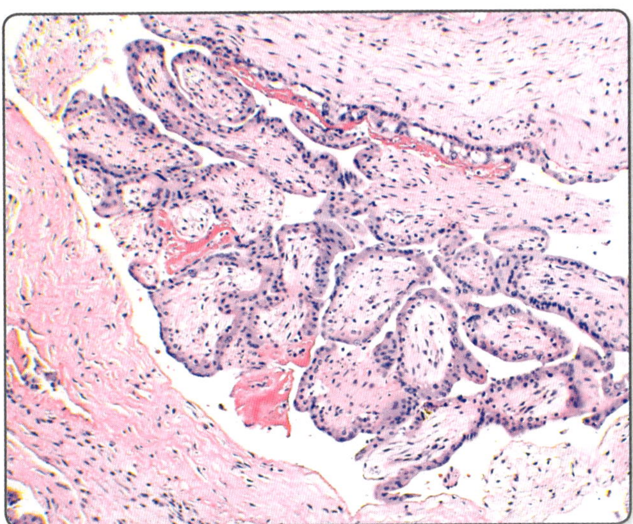

Figure 3.8 Avascular villi may reflect a missed abortion, but may also be seen in pregnancies less than 7–8 weeks.

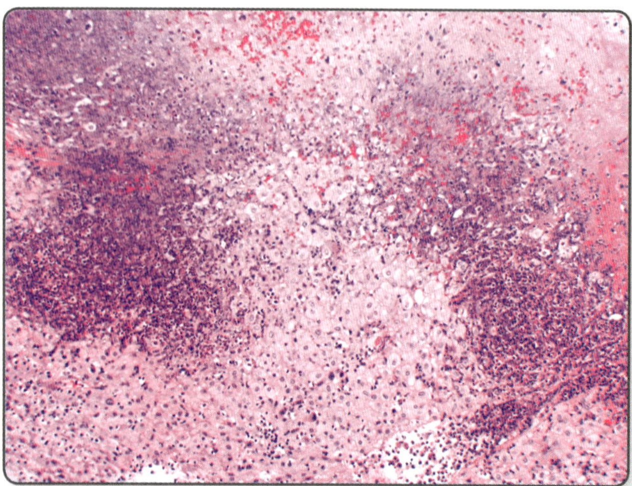

Figure 3.9 Decidua showing necrosis and influx of inflammatory cells.

starts to break down after death of the pregnancy, with influx of inflammatory cells, particularly neutrophils. This does not reflect infective endometritis, but is a mark of inflammation.

Remote from the pregnancy, products of conception may be retained, including retained placental membranes (**Figure 3.10**) or ghost villi (**Figure 3.11a**). These retain the general larger configuration of earlier villi, as opposed to the smaller more agglutinated villi of the third trimester placental polyp (**Figure 3.11b**). The endometrium may begin to cycle again. Chronic endometritis, with plasma cells, may sometimes be seen in these cases.

There have been studies looking at whether chromosomal abnormalities can be predicted by histology, because many first trimester pregnancy losses are due to chromosomal abnormalities, most

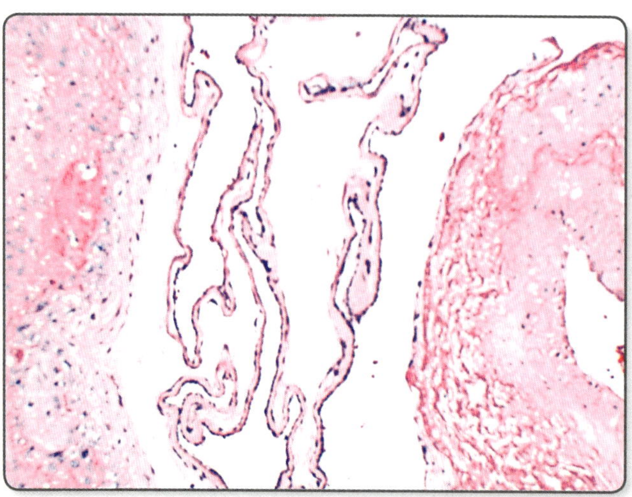

Figure 3.10 Retained fetal membranes.

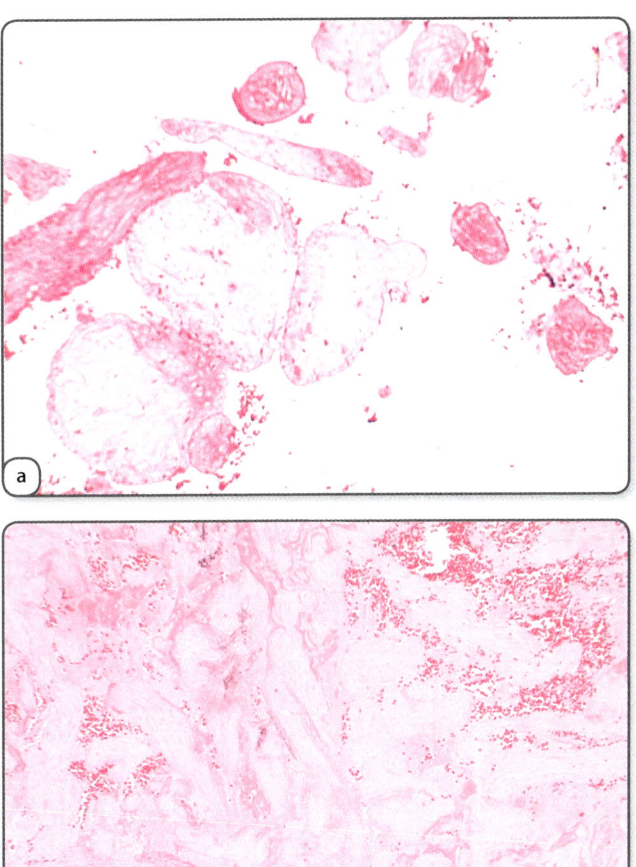

Figure 3.11 Retained necrotic "ghost" chorionic villi is shown in (a). Placental polyp (b) showing agglutinated necrotic third trimester villi.

often triploidy. Triploid pregnancies may show abundant trophoblast inclusions (**Figure 3.12**), however the finding of trophoblast inclusions does not confirm triploidy or other chromosomal abnormality.[4,5]

One of the clinical issues that can arise is when a patient presents with pain, bleeding and positive pregnancy test and the diagnosis is ectopic pregnancy. If there are no intrauterine villi, the differential diagnoses are a complete abortion, i.e. passage of all the products of conception, or an ectopic pregnancy. The implantation site should be sought in these curettage specimens, because this confirms that the pregnancy was intrauterine, effectively ruling out an ectopic pregnancy (unless heterotopic pregnancy is present, an extremely rare occurrence). The implantation site is characterized by Nitabuch's fibrin layer, and implantation trophoblasts. Syncytiotrophoblasts may be seen at the interface, and intermediate trophoblasts may be seen infiltrating the decidua (**Figure 3.13**).

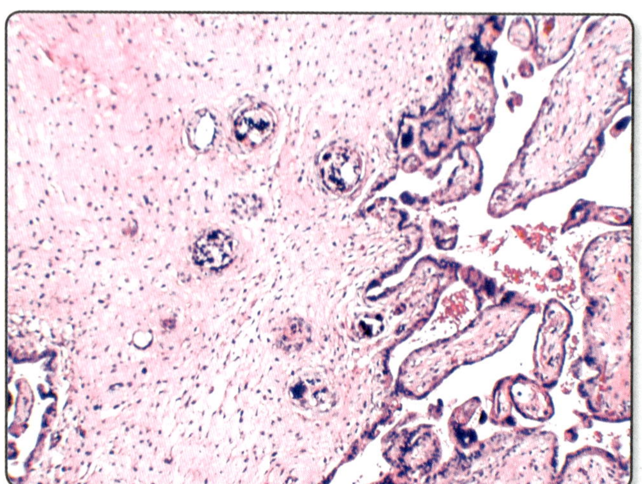

Figure 3.12 Trophoblast inclusions. Scalloped irregular villi cut on edge in sections show what appear to be inclusions. Numerous inclusions are sometimes associated with chromosomal abnormalities, particularly triploidy, but this is not confirmatory.

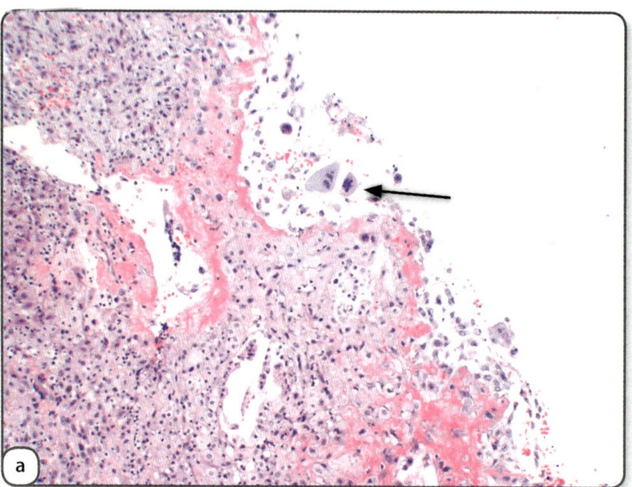

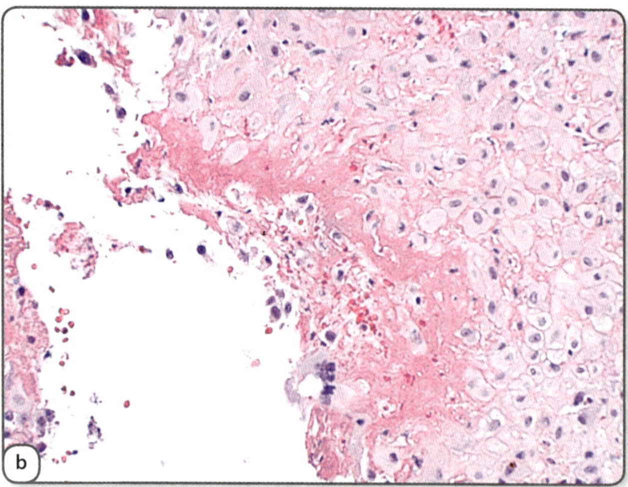

Figure 3.13 Implantation site. (a) Syncytiotrophoblasts (arrow) may be seen above the Nitabuch's fibrin layer. (b) Nitabuch's fibrin layer on the surface of decidua should prompt a search for implantation trophoblasts.

The presence of fibrin material alone is insufficient to confirm an implantation site.

Endometrium associated with ectopic pregnancy

The endometrium associated with an extrauterine pregnancy may have just about any appearance, including proliferative, secretory, or hypersecretory (with or without Arias-Stella reaction). Since ectopic pregnancies outgrow their blood supply and may become nonviable, degenerative changes may be seen as well, including sloughing with breakdown or an involutional secretory pattern (**Figure 3.14**) which is not specifically diagnostic of ectopic pregnancy.

Third trimester endometrial findings

Retained placenta

Retention of placental tissue can lead to bleeding and infection, and thus may be picked up shortly after the pregnancy. Here, the tissue resembles third-trimester placenta with variable degrees of degenerative changes and inflammation. Occasionally the tissue is retained asymptomatically for longer periods of time, in which case ghost villi may be seen. At times a "placental polyp" (see **Figure 3.11b**) may form, a polypoid aggregate of degenerated placental villous tissue, which may be associated with delayed hemorrhage.

Placenta accreta

Placenta accreta has become more common with the increased utilization of Cesarean deliveries. Placenta accreta is the abnormal attachment of the placenta directly to the myometrium, without intervening decidua (**Figure 3.15**). This eliminates the cleavage plane normally present, by which part of the decidua is attached to the

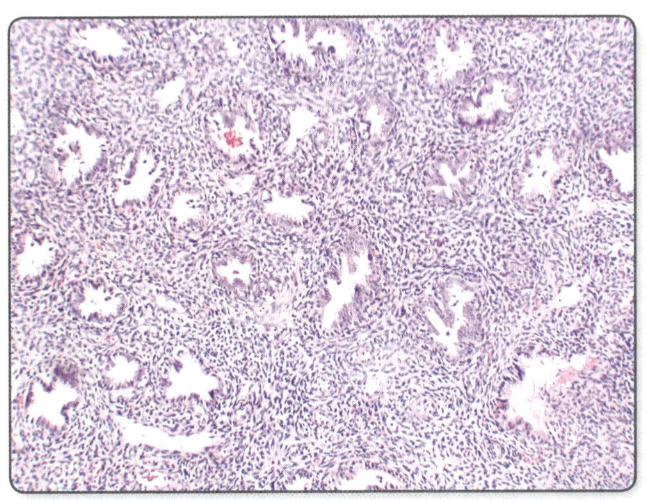

Figure 3.14 **Involuting secretory endometrium** is one pattern that may be seen with an ectopic pregnancy.

delivering placenta and the basal portion remains to regenerate new endometrium. Histologically, it may take many uterine sections to confirm accreta, due to the irregularity of the interface, focality of the lesion (at times), and presence of abundant fibrin. Clinical attempts to remove the placenta may also interfere with the histologic diagnosis.

Risk factors for accreta include prior cesarean sections, or curettages, where the endometrium may be defective. Accreta is a condition that usually presents with postpartum hemorrhage in the third trimester, but it can be seen earlier. If the placental tissue invades into the myometrium, it is called *increta*, and if it penetrates the entire uterine wall, *percreta* (**Figure 3.15b**). Rarely, accreta may be diagnosed from the placenta itself, if sufficient muscle tissue is adherent, but this is rare.

With the increasing use of cesarean section deliveries, there has also been an increase in the number of cases of placenta percreta, and laboratories may notice an increase in cesarean hysterectomy specimens received.

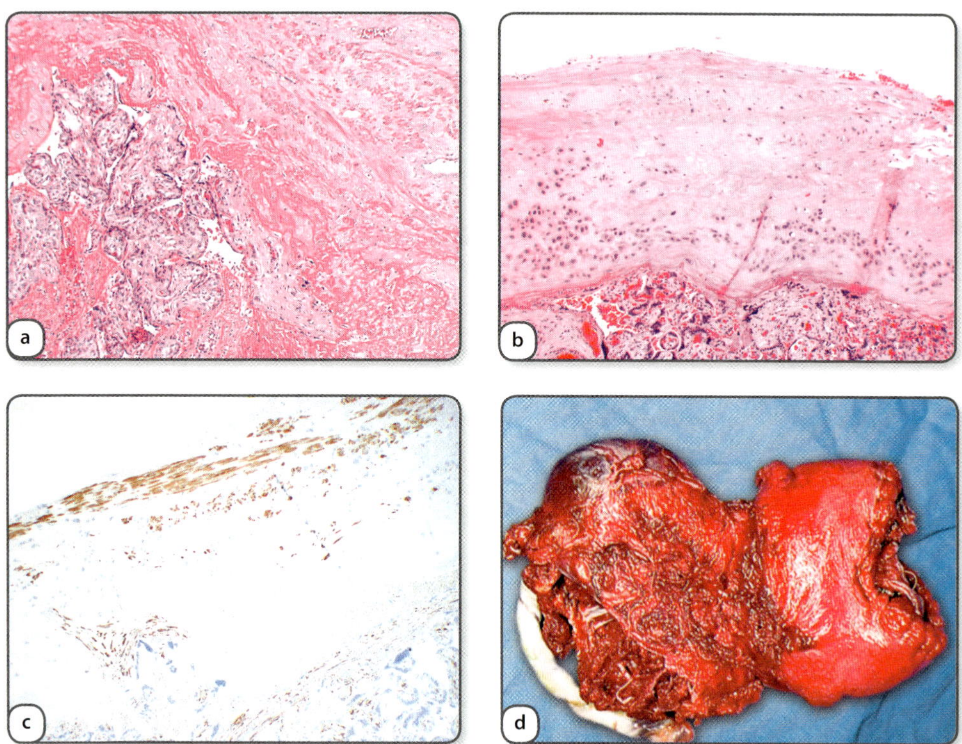

Figure 3.15 Placenta accreta (a), with placental villi in direct contact with myometrium, without the normally intervening decidua. Rarely, muscle fibers can be appreciated on the placenta (b), highlighted by immunostaining for smooth muscle actin (c). Placenta percreta (d), with placental tissue extending through the wall of the myometrium.

Gestational trophoblastic neoplasia (GTN)

Hydatidiform mole

Hydatidiform moles used to be easier to identify histologically, in the era prior to the liberal use of ultrasound in pregnancy, because the molar pregnancies were diagnosed at a later gestational age. The classic clinical picture of a woman with a complete mole with a massively enlarged uterus, who is passing "grapes" per vagina, is not often seen nowadays.

The diagnosis of molar pregnancy is important, as patients need follow-up of their beta human chorionic gonadotropin (bhCG) levels to make sure they don't develop persistent trophoblastic neoplasia. The risk of neoplasia is greater with a complete mole than with a partial mole, hence the distinction is important even though the clinical follow-up is the same. The risk is approximately 0.2–5.0% with partial mole, versus 15–25% with complete mole.[6] Of patients with complete mole, 3–5% goes on to develop choriocarcinoma, which is rare after a partial mole.[6]

Because of the need for extended follow-up, with avoidance of a pregnancy during follow-up (to avoid confusion in interpreting bhCG levels), distinguishing a molar pregnancy from a hydropic missed abortion is also important. The distinction of partial mole from hydropic abortion can be particularly problematic, as will be discussed below. While some cases will be easily diagnosed, ancillary testing may be needed (see p. 41).

Complete hydatidiform mole

Complete moles show a uniformity of abnormal villi. The villi are enlarged, avascular, and hydropic, often to the point of cistern formation in the center. Trophoblast proliferation is diffuse around villi, unlike the polar capping of normal gestations, and is greater in amount than in partial mole. Clusters of extravillous trophoblast may also be seen. Atypia of the trophoblast may be prominent. Complete moles are generally diploid, containing two sets of paternal chromosomal material and no maternal material, due to fertilization of an empty ovum by two spermatozoa or fertilization of one empty ovum with splitting (diandric diploidy).

Early complete hydatidiform moles may not show as prominent edema and trophoblast proliferation, but may instead demonstrate more subtle abnormalities, including bulbous villi, with basophilic hypercellular stroma showing increased apoptosis and at times labyrinthine vessels (**Figures 3.16–3.19**)[7].

Partial hydatidiform mole

Partial moles are usually triploid, with two sets of chromosomes of paternal origin and one maternal (diandric triploidy). Digynic triploid gestations, with two maternal chromosomes and one paternal, give rise to dysmorphic growth retarded fetuses with small placentas.[8]

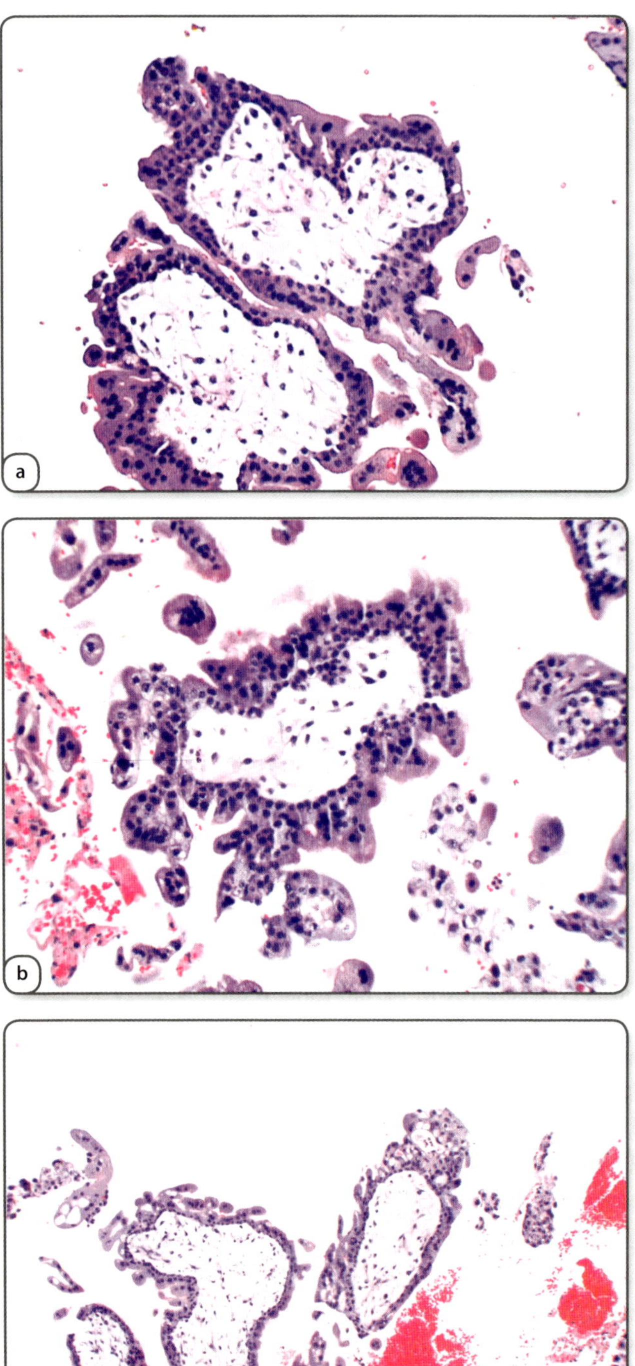

Figure 3.19 Early complete hydatidiform mole showing bulbous villi with hypercellular stroma and circumferential trophoblast proliferation.

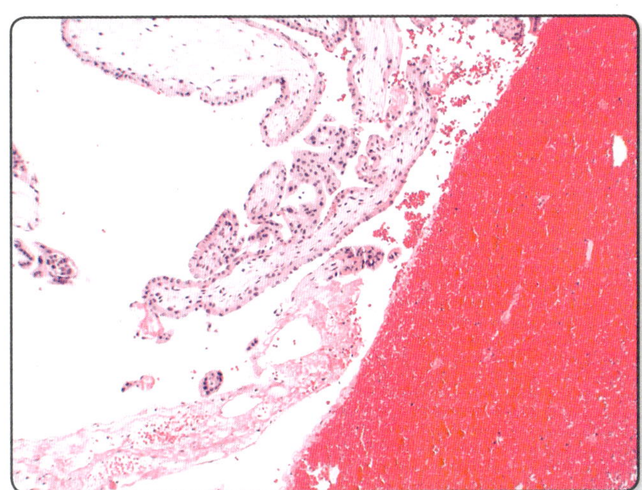

Figure 3.20 Partial mole. Irregular villi with less prominent trophoblast proliferation.

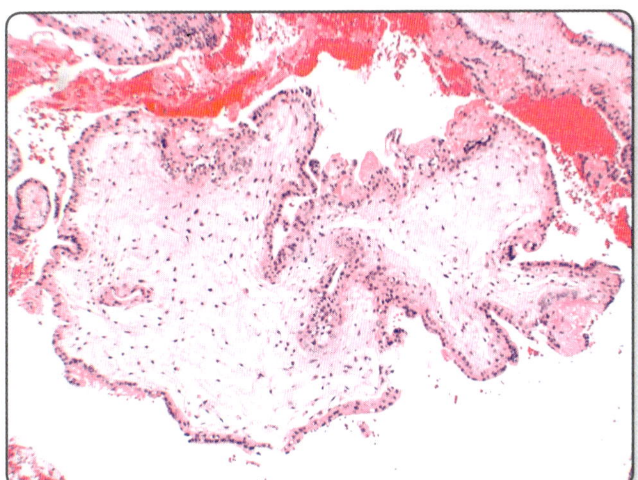

Figure 3.21 Partial mole. Villi may be dysmorphic, with irregular scalloped shapes and trophoblast inclusions.

imaging studies. Rarely are surgical specimens received by pathology laboratories nowadays. GTD may follow a prior hydatidiform mole in about half the cases,[8] but it may also follow a prior term gestation, early pregnancy loss or ectopic pregnancy, and there are clinical criteria for determining risk factors and prognosis as well as stage. Rarely, a uterine specimen may be received with an invasive mole. Histologically, the tissue meets the criteria of a hydatidiform mole, but it is present within the myometrium. It is the presence of the molar villi, in addition to trophoblast proliferation, that distinguishes this entity from choriocarcinoma. In almost all cases, the moles are complete moles.[8]

Gestational choriocarcinoma

Gestational choriocarcinoma is a biphasic neoplasm consisting of multinucleated syncytiotrophoblasts and well-demarcated

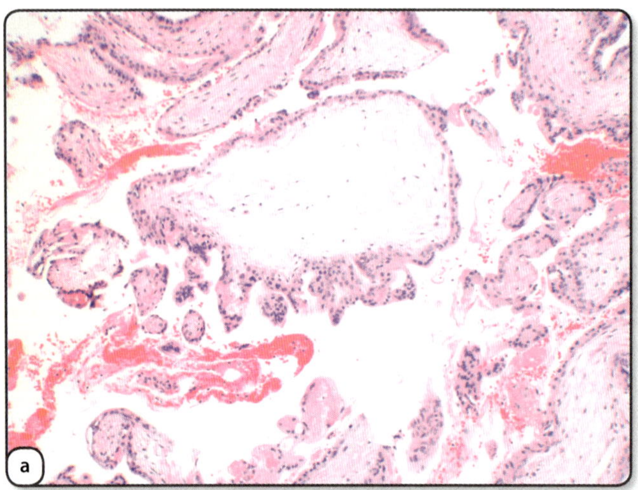

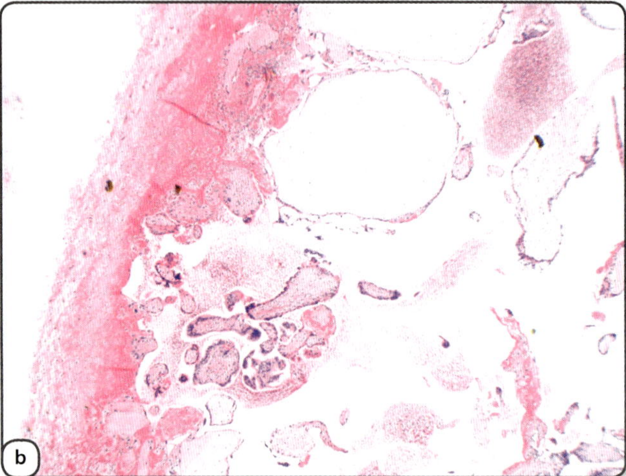

Figure 3.22 Partial mole. A mix of enlarged and normal size villi is seen. Edema and trophoblast proliferation are less pronounced than complete mole.

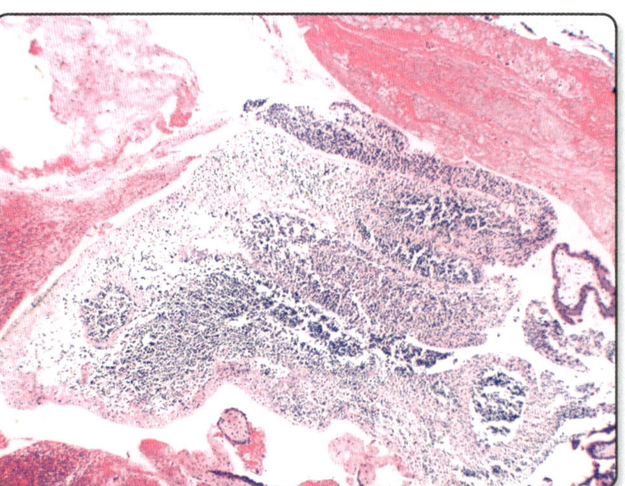

Figure 3.23 Partial mole showing degenerating fetal tissue.

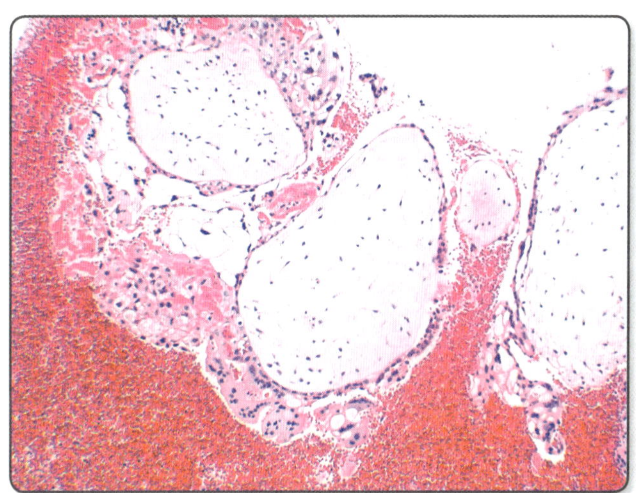

Figure 3.24 Hydatidiform mole. Sometimes distinguishing a complete from a partial mole is difficult on histology. p57 immunostaining was consistent with partial mole.

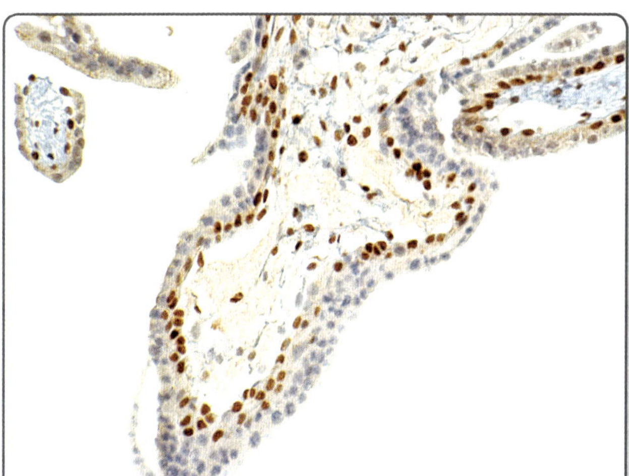

Figure 3.25 Partial mole. p57 immunohistochemistry shows staining of cytotrophoblast and villous mesenchymal cells.

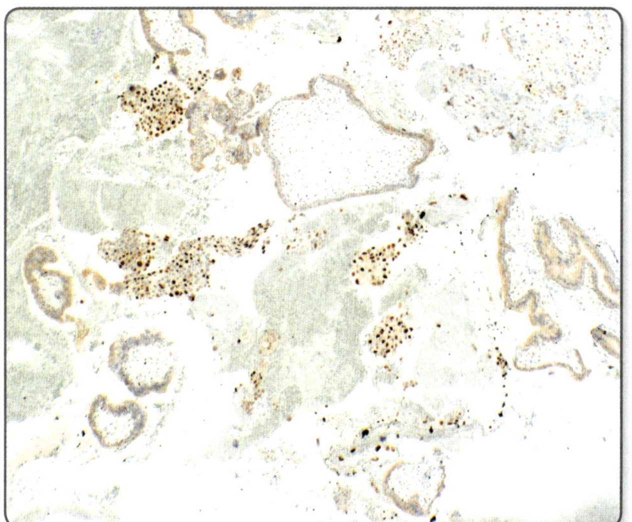

Figure 3.26 Complete mole. p57 immunohistochemistry shows staining of extravillous trophoblast, but no staining of villi is seen.

cytotrophoblasts, often with prominent atypia. The syncytiotrophoblasts will stain for hCG by immunohistochemistry.[8] The neoplasm is extremely hemorrhagic. It is occasionally detected on a curettage specimen, but is often a biopsy specimen from an extrauterine location, if any tissue is submitted at all (**Figures 3.27** and **3.28**).

Placental site trophoblastic tumor (PSTT)

Placental site trophoblastic tumor is a lesion of intermediate trophoblasts. Although it can be suspected on a curettage specimen, it is usually diagnosed at hysterectomy. The patients usually have been pregnant at some point in their lives, but the timing may have been remote from the PSTT. BhCG is elevated, but only moderately. The lesions are composed of intermediate trophoblast cells, which infiltrate into the myometrium. The cells stain for human placental

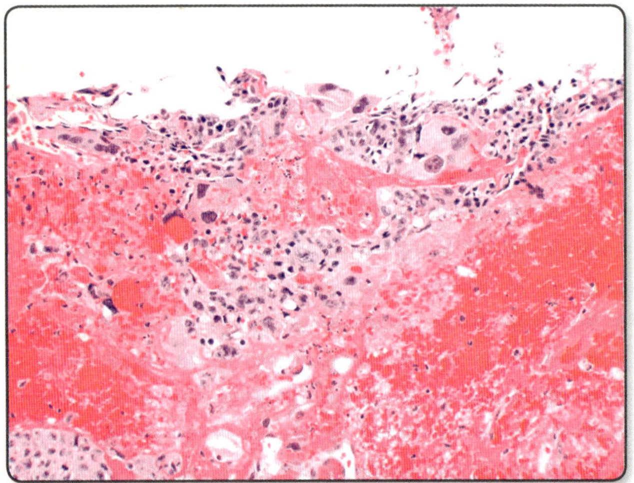

Figure 3.27 Choriocarcinoma. Clusters of biphasic tumor cells are seen within blood clot, in this extremely hemorrhagic tumor.

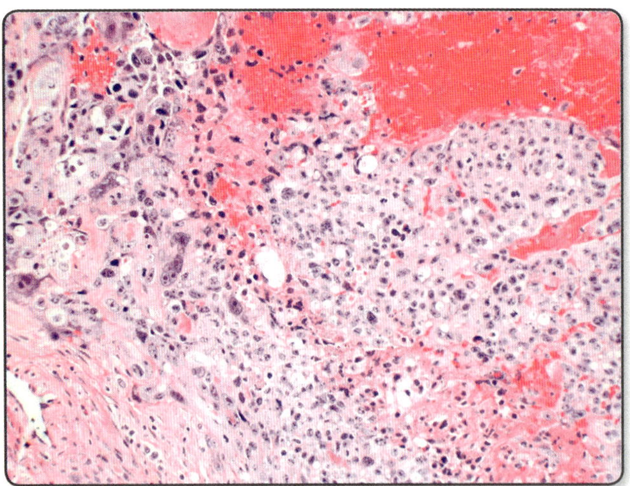

Figure 3.28 Choriocarcinoma. The biphasic nature of the tumor can be appreciated.

lactogen, and only mildly or focally for human chorionic gonadotropin (HCG). The splitting of myometrial bundles is characteristic. The intermediate trophoblast cells are usually mononuclear, but may be binuclear (**Figures 3.29** and **3.30**). The lesion appears similar to but more exuberant than an exaggerated implantation site, with which it may be confused (see p. 48). PSTT usually forms a mass, in contrast to exaggerated implantation site. PSTT is usually treated by hysterectomy and behaves in a benign fashion in most cases, but up to 15% of the tumors show malignant behavior.[8]

Epithelioid trophoblastic tumor (ETT)

This rare and recently described tumor of extravillous intermediate trophoblast is thought to resemble and possibly arise from the trophoblasts of the chorion laeve.[10,11] Thus, the lesion is nodular, as is

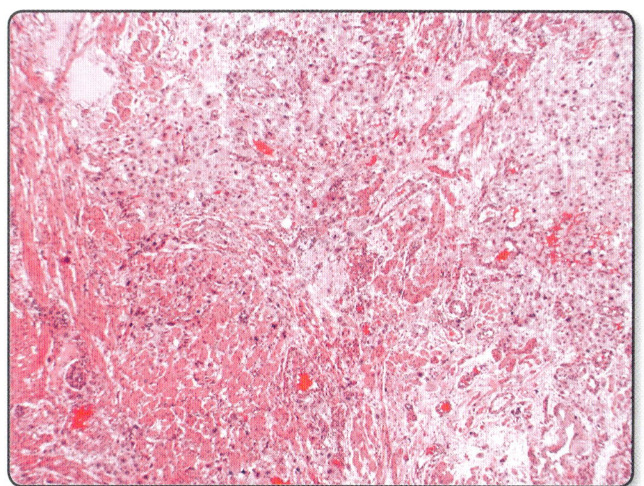

Figure 3.29 Placental site trophoblastic tumor. The tumor cells are seen splitting the myometrial bundles.

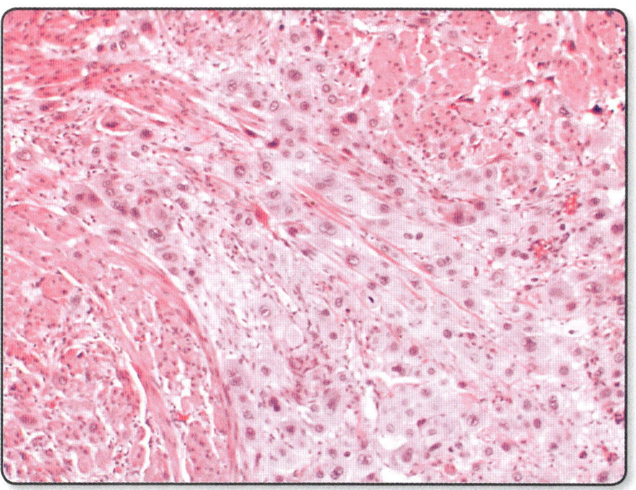

Figure 3.30 Placental site trophoblastic tumor at higher power, the tumor cells infiltrating between the myometrium are intermediate trophoblasts, predominantly with single nuclei.

the originating trophoblast of the chorion, in contrast to PSTT, which is infiltrative, as is its putative cytotrophoblast of origin, the implantation trophoblast.[11] The clinical history is similar to PSTT, with pregnancy often a remote event.

Histologically, the cells are a nodular monomorphic population of intermediate trophoblast cells with abundant eosinophilic cytoplasm and hyaline material. Positive human placental lactogen (hPL), cytokeratin-18 (CK-18) and inhibin staining will help distinguish the lesion from a squamous cell lesion (a possible differential due to the eosinophilic material, as well as the fact that ETT stains for cytokeratins and p63, similar to squamous cell carcinoma).[11] Adding to the difficulty of this distinction is the propensity of ETT to arise in the lower uterine segment or endocervix.[11] Its cyclin E index is much higher than in placental site nodules[10,11], also in the differentials, but it has a higher Ki-67 proliferation index than placental site nodules.[11] ETT can be distinguished from PSTT by the more infiltrative nature of PSTT, with more vascular invasion, as well as greater hPL positivity in PSTT. PSTT is also shows greater positivity for Mel-CAM, and is negative for p63, distinguishing it from ETT.[11] The behavior and metastatic potential of ETT appear similar to PSTT.[12,13]

Trophoblastic lesions that may be confused with GTN

Exaggerated placental site

Exaggerated placental site is the lesion most likely to be confused with a PSTT, particularly on curettage specimens. It can be seen on curettage specimens associated with a current or recent pregnancy. Since the uterus is very soft during pregnancy, curettage may yield fragments of myometrium showing similar intermediate trophoblast cells to PSTT (**Figure 3.31**). The clinical picture is usually different, with a current

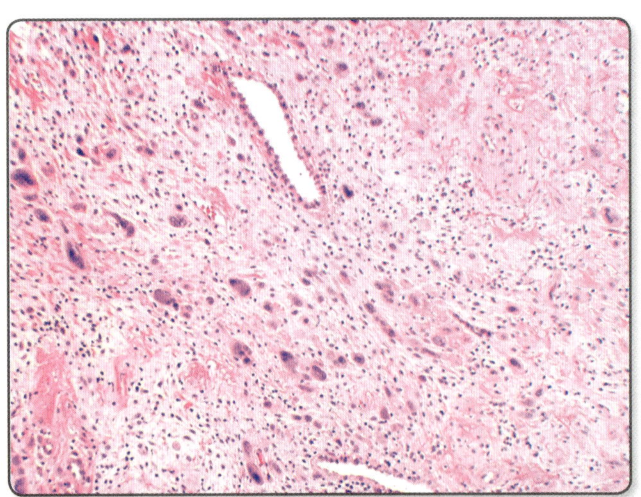

Figure 3.31 Exaggerated placental site showing numerous intermediate trophoblasts in decidua. These also extend into myometrium, sometimes raising concern for a placental site trophoblastic tumor.

pregnancy with significantly elevated bhCG, as opposed to the low bhCG of PSTT. A Ki-67 proliferation index of <1% favors exaggerated placental site, while >10% favors PSTT.[8]

Placental site nodules and plaques

Placental site nodules and plaques are usually incidental findings, the hallmark of a remote pregnancy. Nodular or plaque-like lesions containing occasional intermediate trophoblasts in a hyalinized background are seen (**Figure 3.32**). The Ki-67 proliferation rate of <10% helps separate it from PSTT, if concern arises.

Persistent gestational trophoblastic disease

The diagnosis of persistent gestational trophoblastic disease after evacuation of a hydatidiform mole is usually a clinical one, supported by a plateau or rise in bhCG titers. It may be further evaluated by imaging studies, however the pathologist rarely receives additional pathologic material. In some cases, curettage may be performed, and it is not always possible to make an exact diagnosis. The curettings shown in **Figure 3.33** are from a patient 4 months postevacuation of a hydatidiform mole. They show rare atypical trophoblast cells in blood clot, but the majority of the specimen was proliferative endometrium. This abnormal focus may represent choriocarcinoma, however it may also represent persistent mole with no villi obtained, or invasive mole with no villi obtained. Additionally, although unlikely, it could represent the remnants of a new gestation, either normal or abnormal. In cases such as these, a descriptive diagnosis is warranted, and it can be stated that this is consistent with the clinical diagnosis of persistent GTD. Staging of gestational trophoblastic neoplasia (**Table 3.1**) is based on predominantly clinical factors.

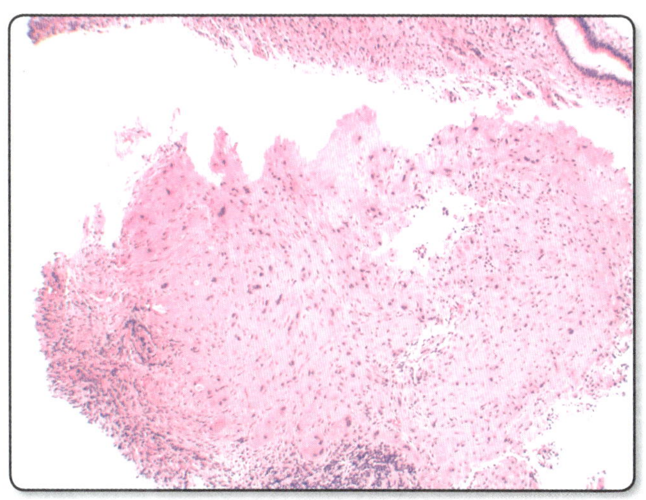

Figure 3.32 Placental site nodule. A nodular endometrial lesion composed of scant intermediate trophoblasts in a hyalinized background.

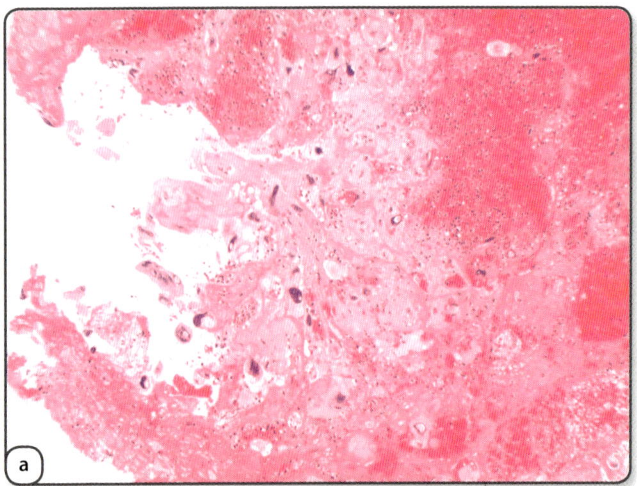

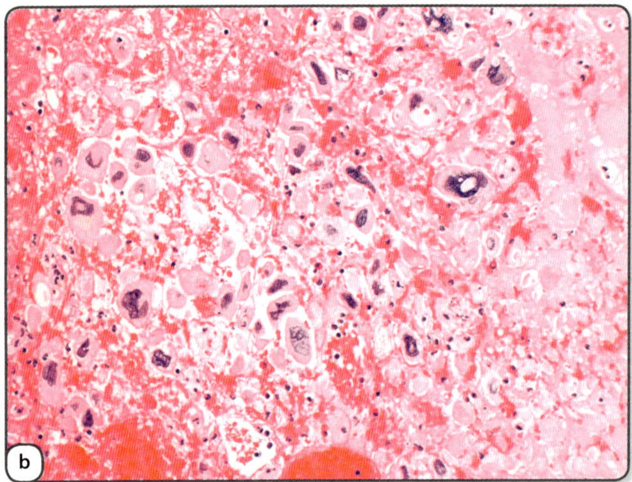

Figure 3.33 Persistent gestational trophoblastic disease. Curettings from a patient with rising hCG titers 4 months after evacuation of a mole.

References

1. Arias-Stella, J. The Arias-Stella reaction: facts and fancies four decades after. Adv Anat Pathol 2002;9:12–23.
2. Vang R, Barner R, Wheeler DT, Strauss BL. Immunohistochemical staining for Ki-67 and p53 helps distinguish endometrial Arias-Stella reaction from high-grade carcinoma, including clear cell carcinoma. Int J. Gynecol Pathol 2004;23:23–33.
3. Simpson JL Causes of fetal wastage. Clin Obstet Gynecol. 2007;50:10–30.
4. Lorenzato M, Visseaux-Coletto B, Lallemand A, Masure M, Gaillard D. Determination of reliable histological features associated with early triploidy using DNA image cytometry. Pathol Res Pract 1995;191:1179–85.
5. Redline RW, Zaragoza M, Hassold T. Prevalence of developmental and inflammatory lesions in nonmolar first-trimester spontaneous abortions. Hum Pathol 1999;30:93–100.
6. Kipp BR, Ketterling RP, Oberg TN, Cousin MA, Plagge AM, Wiktor AE et al. Comparison of fluorescence in situ hybridization, p57 immunostaining, flow cytometry, and digital image analysis for diagnosing molar and nonmolar products of conception. Am J Clin Pathol 2010;133:196–204.

Gestational trophoblastic neoplasia				
FIGO anatomical staging				
Stage I	Disease confined to the uterus			
Stage II	GTN extends outside of the uterus, but is limited to the genital structures (adnexa, vagina, broad ligament)			
Stage III	GTN extends to the lungs, with or without known genital tract involvement			
Stage IV	All other metastatic sites			
Modified WHO prognostic scoring system (as adapted by FIGO)				
Scores	**0**	**1**	**2**	**4**
Age	<40	≥40	n/a	n/a
Antecedent pregnancy	mole	abortion	term	
Interval months from index pregnancy	<4	4–6	7–12	>12
Pretreatment serum hCG (iu/L)	$<10^3$	10^3–10^4	10^4–10^5	$>10^5$
Largest tumor size (including uterus)	<3	3–4	≥5 cm	n/a
Site of metastases	lung	spleen, kidney	gastrointestinal	liver, brain
Number of metastases	n/a	1–4	5–8	>8
Previous failed chemotherapy	n/a	n/a	single drug	2 or more drugs

Table 3.1 Gestational trophoblastic neoplasia. Revised FIGO staging and modified WHO Prognostic Scoring System as Adapted by FIGO. Reprinted from *International Journal of Gynecology & Obstetrics,* volume 105 number 1, FIGO staging for cancer of the vagina, fallopian tube, ovary, and gestational trophoblastic neoplasia, p.3–4, 2009 with permission from Elsevier.

7. Kim KR, Park BH, Hong YO, Kwon HC, Robboy SJ The villous stromal constituents of complete hydatidiform mole differ histologically in very early pregnancy from the normally developing placenta. Am J Surg Pathol. 2009;33:176–85.
8. Hui P. Martel M. Parkash V. Gestational trophoblastic diseases: recent advances in histopathologic diagnosis and related genetic aspects. Adv Anat Pathol 2005;12:116–25.
9. Castrillon DH. Sun D. Weremowicz S. Fisher RA. Crum CP. Genest DR Discrimination of complete hydatidiform mole from its mimics by immunohistochemistry of the paternally imprinted gene product p57 KIP2. Am J Surg Pathol 2001; 25:1225–30.
10. Wells M. The pathology of gestational trophoblastic disease: recent advances. Pathology. 2007;39:88–96.
11. Allison KH, Love JE, Garcia RL Epithelioid trophoblastic tumor: review of a rare neoplasm of the chorionic-type intermediate trophoblast. Arch Pathol Lab Med. 2006;130:1875–77.
12. Shih IM, Kurman RJ. Epithelioid trophoblastic tumor: a neoplasm distinct from choriocarcinoma and placental site trophoblastic tumor simulating carcinoma. Am J Surg Pathol 1998; 22:1393–1403.
13. Shih, I. M. and R. J. Kurman . The pathology of intermediate trophoblastic tumors and tumor-like lesions. Int J Gynecol Pathol 2001;20:31–47.

4 Organic lesions of the endometrium

It should be remembered that bleeding perceived as uterine bleeding by the patient may be due to genital tract disease of other organs, including infections or neoplasms of cervix, vagina, or fallopian tubes,[1] or may be due to nongenital causes, such as bleeding from the rectum or bladder. Causes of uterine bleeding due to intrinsic uterine pathology are termed *organic*. This chapter focuses on the pathology associated with intrinsic uterine disease leading to abnormal bleeding.

Endometrial polyps

Usual endometrial polyps

Endometrial polyps may be silent, but they often manifest as intermenstrual spotting or postmenopausal bleeding. Histologically, the intact endometrial polyp is a straightforward diagnosis. The lesion is polypoid in shape, and covered by an endometrial-type epithelial lining. The stroma is more fibrous than the surrounding endometrial stroma, hence more eosinophilic. Large, thick stalk vessels may be seen. The glands are usually nonsecretory, showing more estrogenic response than progesterone response; hence they often appear as simple hyperplasia within the polyp (**Figures 4.1–4.3**). If the specimen also includes nonpolyp endometrium, the lack of simple hyperplasia in that endometrium will demonstrate the distinction. However, if there is no adjacent endometrium in the sample, and the polyps are fragmented, it may be difficult to rule out simple hyperplasia.

It is known that in-office biopsies may miss focal lesions such as polyps, and these patients may require curettage. Endometrial polyps are often fragmented by the curettage procedure, and it becomes more challenging to confirm the diagnosis when not all characteristic histologic features have been preserved. However, if adjacent endometrium is sampled, it may be of different phase than the presumed polyp, aiding in the distinction. A diagnosis of "probable endometrial polyp", coupled with the clinical impression based on history, examination, and adjunct studies such as imaging, will satisfactorily confirm the presence of a polyp (**Figures 4.4** and **4.5**).

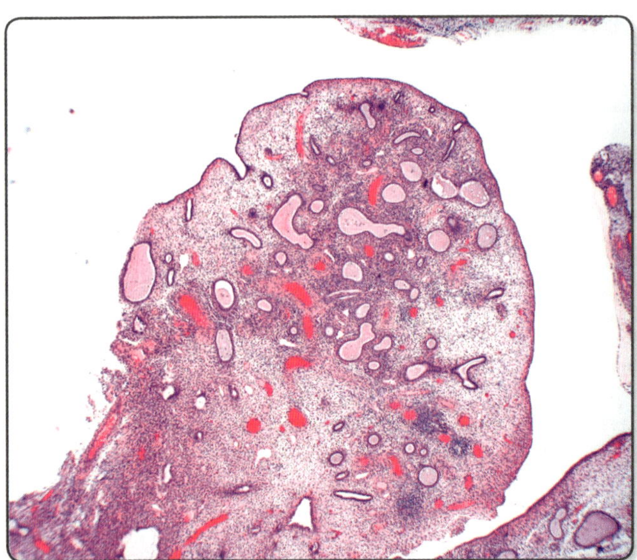

Figure 4.1 Endometrial polyp. At low power, the intact polyp may be seen to have a polypoid shape, with cystically dilated glands. Thick stalk vessels may be seen

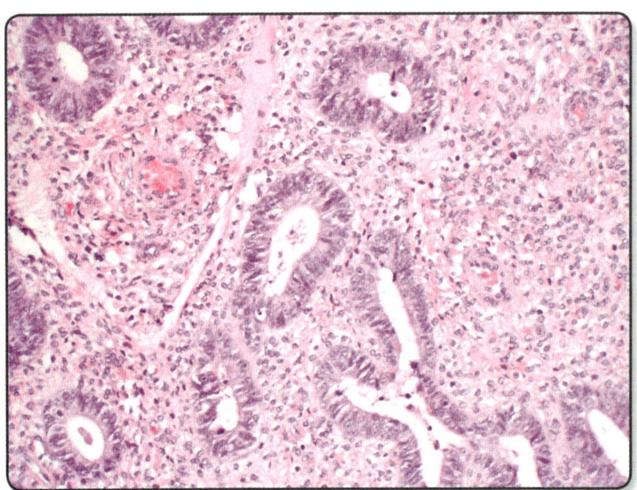

Figure 4.2 Endometrial polyp. Irregular nonsecretory glands are seen

Aside from causing bleeding, the question arises as to whether there is any malignant potential in an endometrial polyp. In a recent meta-analysis, malignancy rates were low, but not absent, with risk factors for malignancy being symptomatic vaginal bleeding and postmenopausal status. In this analysis, premalignant or malignant changes were present in 5.42% of postmenopausal women (versus 1.7% of premenopausal women) and in 4.15% of symptomatic women (versus 2.16% of women without bleeding).[2]

Adenomyomatous polyps

A variant of usual endometrial polyp, the adenomyomatous polyp contains variable amounts of smooth muscle in the stroma. This is a

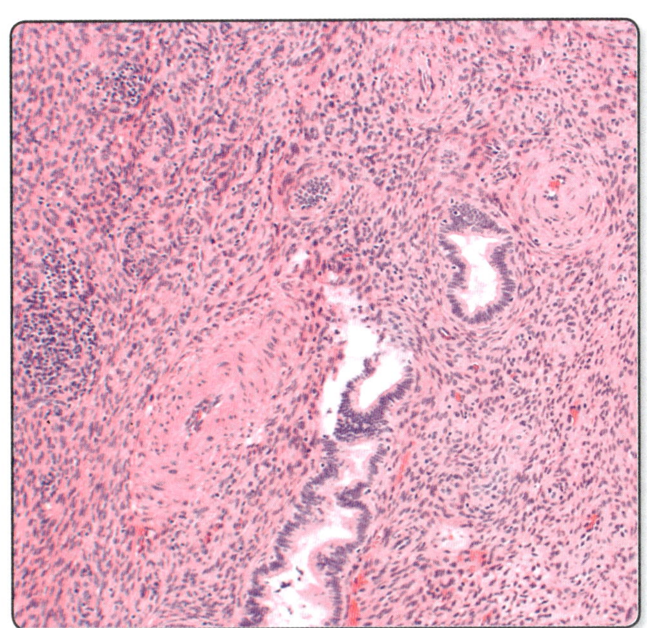

Figure 4.3 Endometrial polyp. Eosinophilic stroma, irregular glands, and thick stalk vessels are seen.

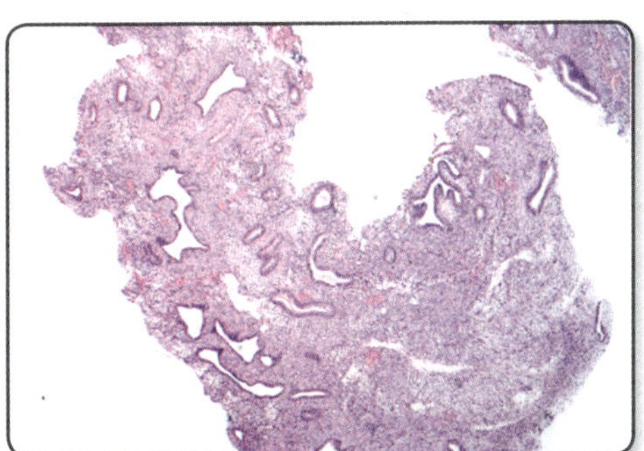

Figure 4.4 Probable endometrial polyp. Irregular glands are seen in a vaguely polypoid fragment, but other diagnostic features are not present.

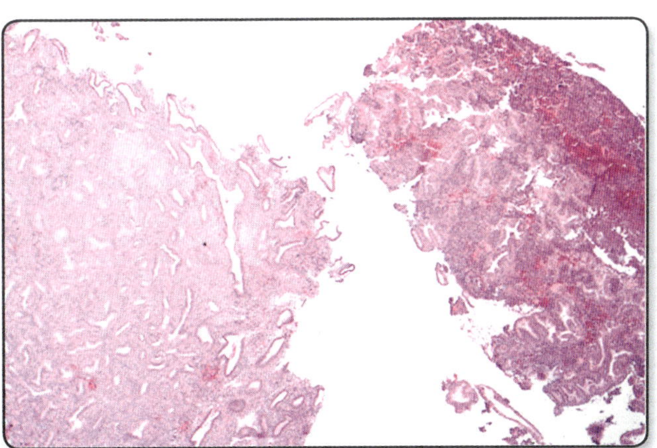

Figure 4.5 Probable endometrial polyp on the left. The right sided fragment shows shedding secretory endometrium. The fact that the probable polyp is in a different phase than surrounding endometrium is supportive of the diagnosis.

histologic variant, and its clinical significance is no different from the usual polyp (**Figure 4.6**). The smooth muscle may be delineated by trichrome stain (**Figure 4.7**) or immunohistochemical markers of smooth muscle, such as smooth muscle actin.

Atypical polypoid adenomyoma (APA)

Atypical polypoid adenomyoma is a rare polypoid lesion arising in the uterus and which occurs most often in women of reproductive age. Hence, although hysterectomy is generally the treatment of choice, uterine-sparing procedures have been utilized. Although initially described as a benign lesion, there is some evidence of an association with endometrial adenocarcinoma, in the range of 8.8% in one literature review.[3]

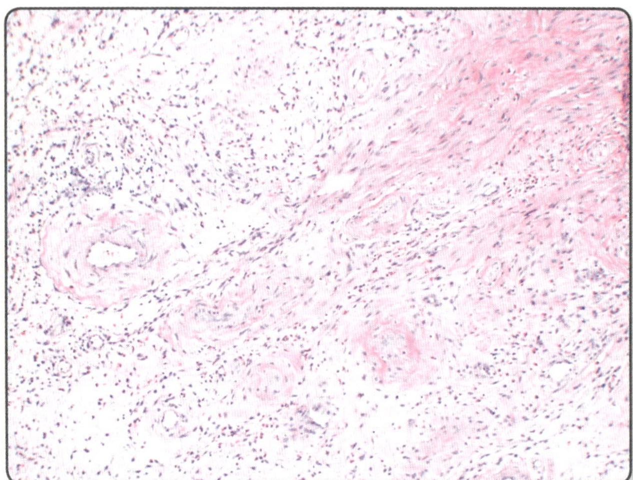

Figure 4.6 Adenomyomatous polyp. Features are similar to a usual endometrial polyp, however bundles of smooth muscle are present in the stroma of the polyp admixed with fibroconnective tissue and thick stalk vessels.

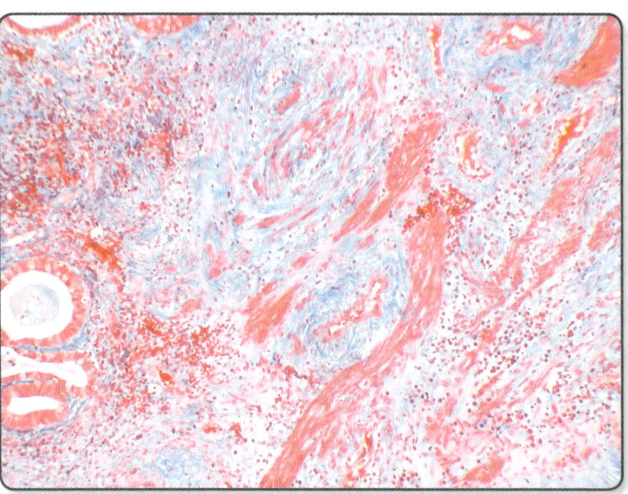

Figure 4.7 Adenomyomatous polyp. The smooth muscle fibers are delineated by trichrome stain, showing red muscle fibers admixed with blue fibroconnective tissue.

Histologically, the lesion is composed of nonsecretory endometrial glands embedded in a benign smooth muscle stroma. The glands may be architecturally complex and cytologically atypical, raising the concern that a myoinvasive endometrial adenocarcinoma may be present. The pathologist may be confronted with making the diagnosis on a curettage specimen, which can be very difficult. Squamous metaplasia in the form of morules is a common finding in the glands (**Figures 4.8–4.10**).

With respect to the most common concern in APA – that the lesion represents an endometrial adenocarcinoma invading myometrium – Ohishi et al[4] have demonstrated a characteristic "fringe-like" staining pattern of CD10 around myoinvasive glands of endometrial adenocarcinoma that is not present in APA.

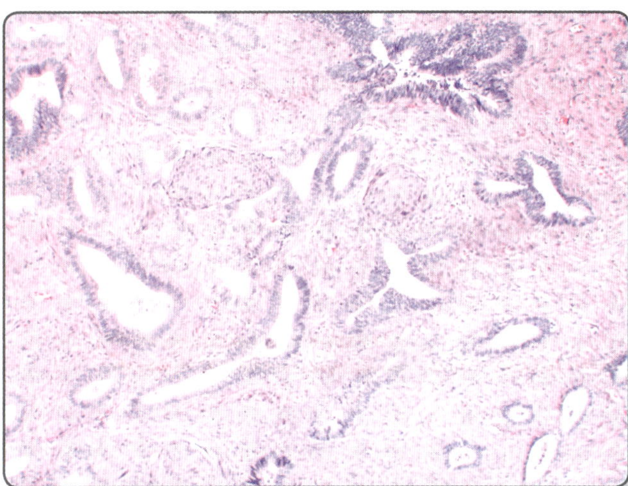

Figure 4.8 Atypical polypoid adenomyoma. Irregular glands in a smooth muscle stroma. Squamous metaplasia is present.

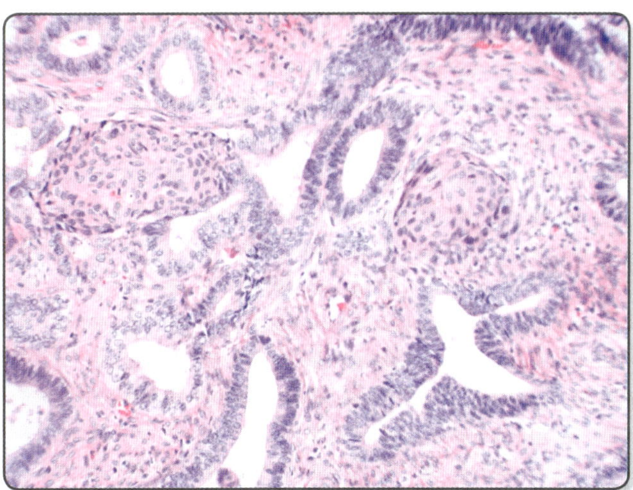

Figure 4.9 Atypical polypoid adenomyoma. At higher power, the characteristic squamous metaplasia is seen.

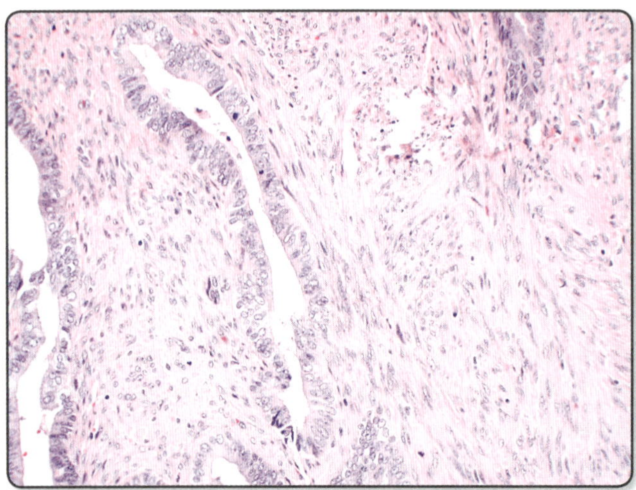

Figure 4.10 Atypical polypoid adenomyoma. Glandular cytologic atypia and mitotic activity, as seen here, may raise the concern of myometrial invasion by an endometrial adenocarcinoma.

Endometritis

Acute endometritis

Acute endometritis is a rare diagnosis, and was more commonly seen in the era of illegal abortions, with postabortal endometritis. Neutrophils are a normal part of the menstrual cycle, so in order to histologically diagnose acute endometritis neutrophils must be seen either within the glandular epithelium or forming microabscesses (**Figures 4.11–4.13**).

Chronic endometritis

Most chronic endometritis does not have a specific identifiable etiology. The histologic hallmark is the plasma cell. Chronic plasmacytic endometritis may be a reactive or infectious condition.[5] It may be associated with disruptions of the morphology of the endometrium,[5] and hence dating in the presence of chronic endometritis should be undertaken with caution, if at all. The condition is included under causes of uterine bleeding here, but chronic endometritis is often an incidental finding, and the association with bleeding is controversial.[6] Plasma cells may be difficult to identify, as endometrial stromal cells may resemble plasma cells. Immunohistochemistry for markers of plasma cells has been attempted. CD38 also stains endometrial glands and stroma, so is not helpful, however it has been demonstrated that CD138 (syndecan) has utility.[7] Plasma cells should be sought particularly if there is irregularity of the glands, or if there are variations in density or increased cellularity of the stroma (**Figures 4.14–4.18**)

Another uncommon variant is xanthogranulomatous endometritis, containing foamy macrophages (**Figure 4.19**). This may be seen in cases of obstruction to endometrial outflow, such as cervical stenosis.[8]

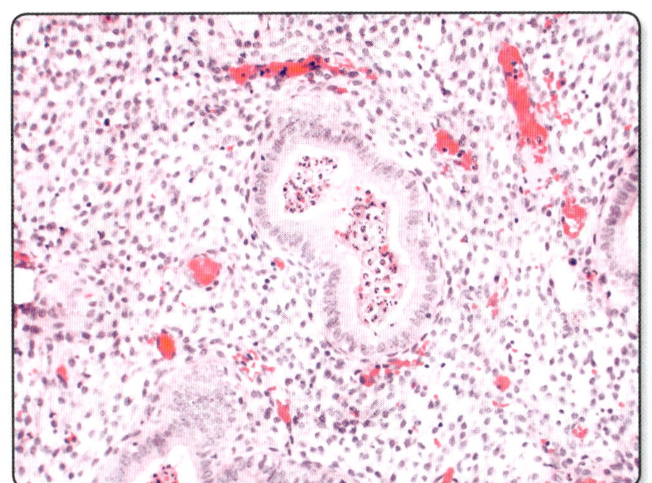

Figure 4.11 Acute endometritis. Numerous neutrophils in glandular lumens

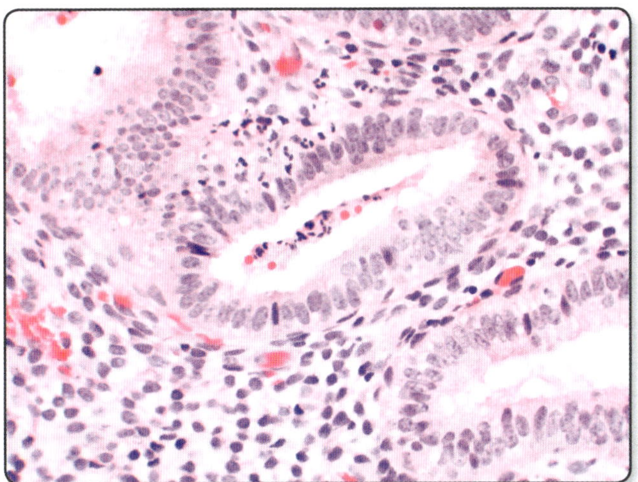

Figure 4.12 Acute endometritis. Neutrophils infiltrating glandular epithelium

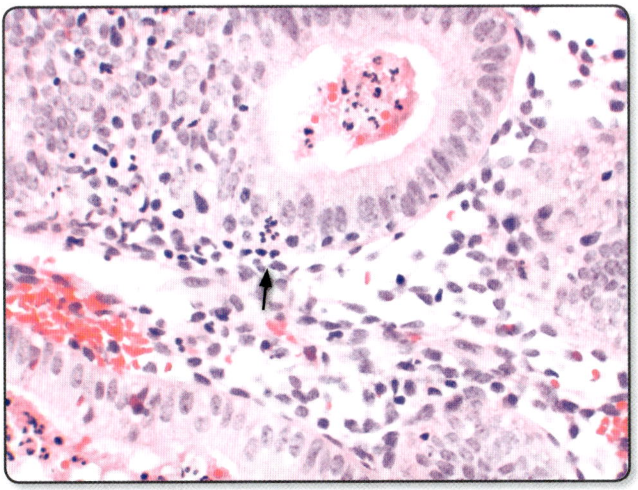

Figure 4.13 Acute endometritis. A small microabscess is seen (arrow).

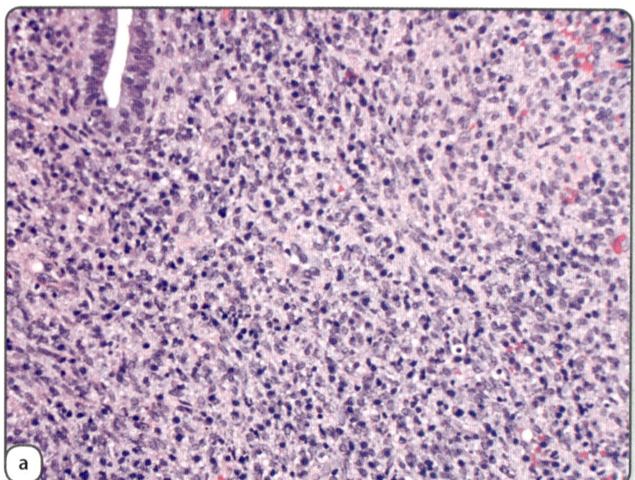

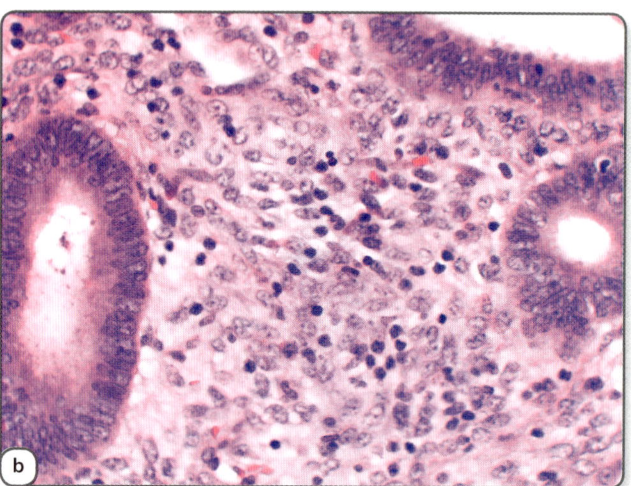

Figure 4.14 Chronic endometritis. The increased cellularity of the stroma should prompt a perusal for plasma cells (a), but the presence of lymphocytes does not signify chronic endometritis (b).

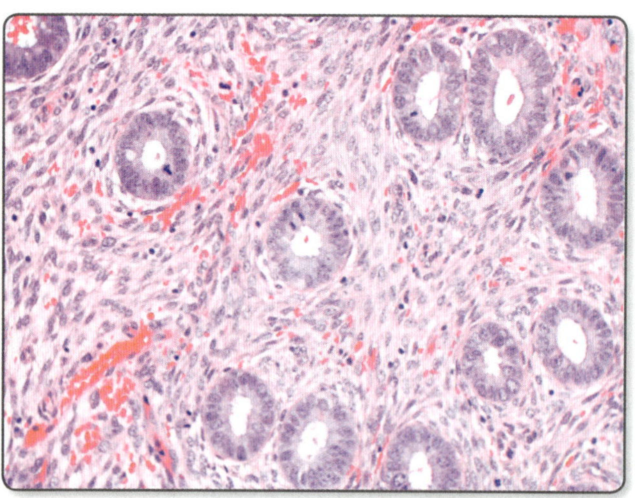

Figure 4.15 Chronic endometritis. The spindling of the stromal cells is another indicator that a scan for plasma cells should be made.

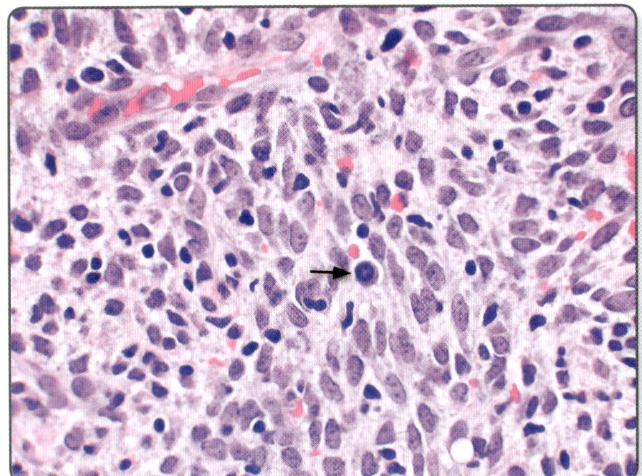

Figure 4.16 Chronic endometritis. Arrow delineates a plasma cell.

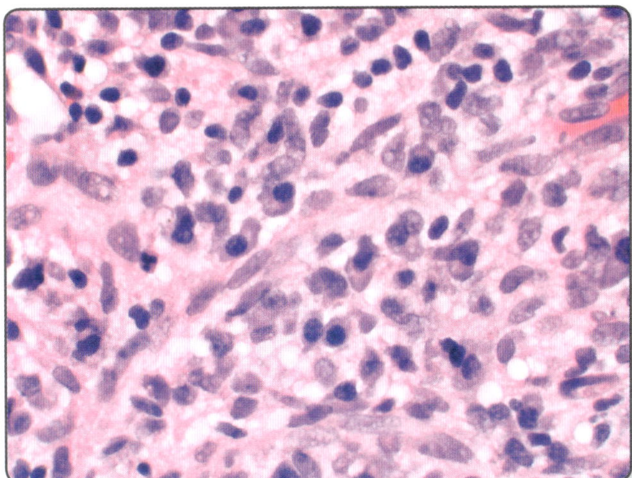

Figure 4.17 Chronic endometritis. Numerous plasma cells are seen, however they may be difficult to distinguish from stromal cells on hematoxylin and eosin stain.

Specific identifiable causes of endometritis

Specific etiologic agents associated with chronic endometritis may rarely be seen. These include tuberculosis, which manifests as granulomatous endometritis. Fungi, schistosomiasis, pinworm and toxoplasma can present as granulomatous endometritis, as can cytomegalovirus and mycoplasma.[9] Noninfectious causes of granulomatous endometritis include sarcoid, reaction to the keratin associated with squamous differentiation, or reaction to foreign materials or associated with endometrial ablation.[9]

Further identifiable causes of chronic endometritis include actinomyces, associated with intrauterine devices, and herpes (**Figures 4.20** and **4.21**). A noninfectious mimic of actinomyces, pseudoactinomycotic granules, containing club-shaped eosinophilic structures radiating

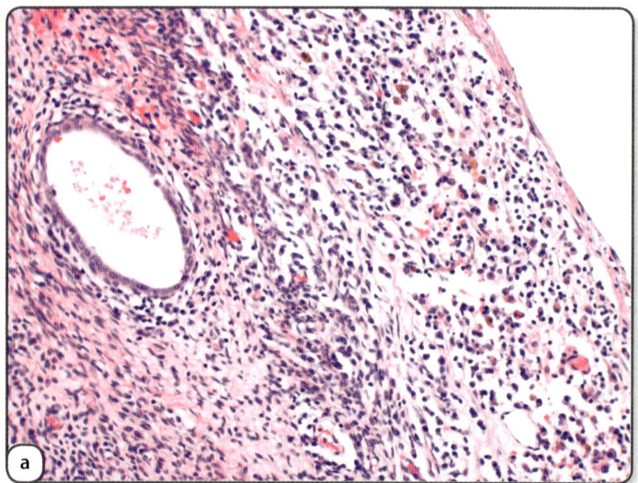

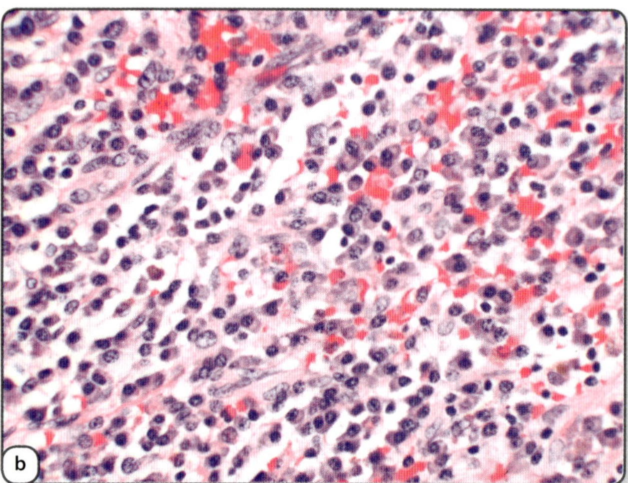

Figure 4.18 Chronic endometritis. The patient had a longstanding history of leiomyomata and pyometra. Note almost complete replacement of the endometrium by plasma cells.

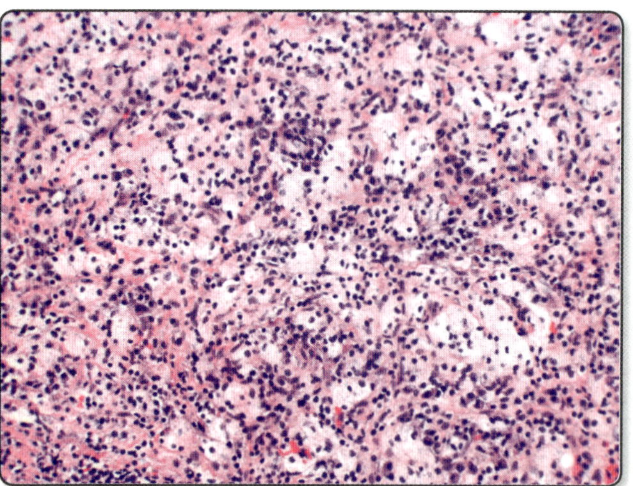

Figure 4.19 Xanthogranulomatous endometritis. Note numerous foamy macrophages admixed with chronic inflammatory cells.

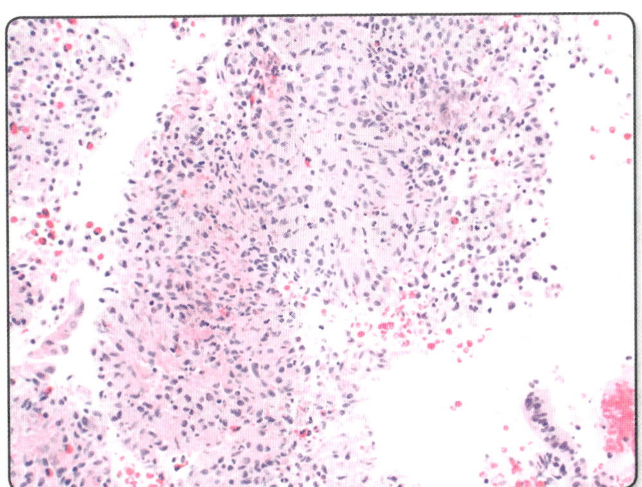

Figure 4.20 Granulomatous endometritis. This may be a manifestation of a variety of infections, including cytomegalovirus or tuberculosis.

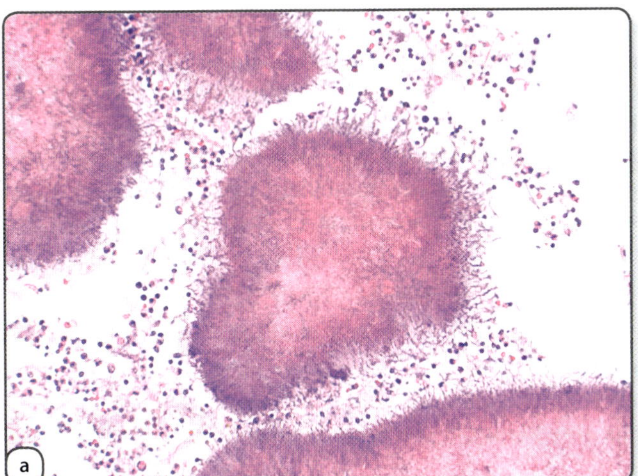

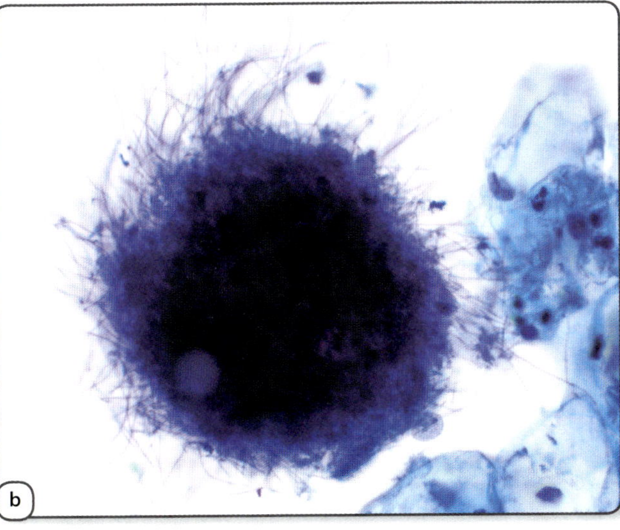

Figure 4.21 Actinomyces. This intrauterine device-associated organism may be seen in association with chronic endometritis. It may be seen on a pap smear (b). The clinician must be notified of the finding, which may require an intervention.

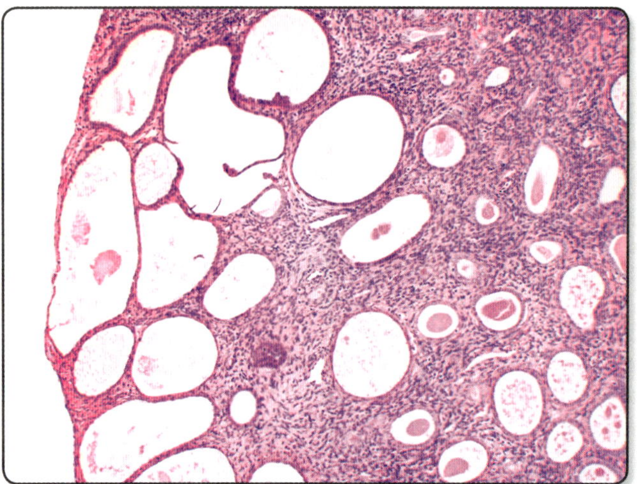

Figure 4.25 Atrophy. On sections from hysterectomies, atrophy may appear as cystic atrophy, distinguished from simple hyperplasia by the flat glandular epithelium lacking mitotic activity.

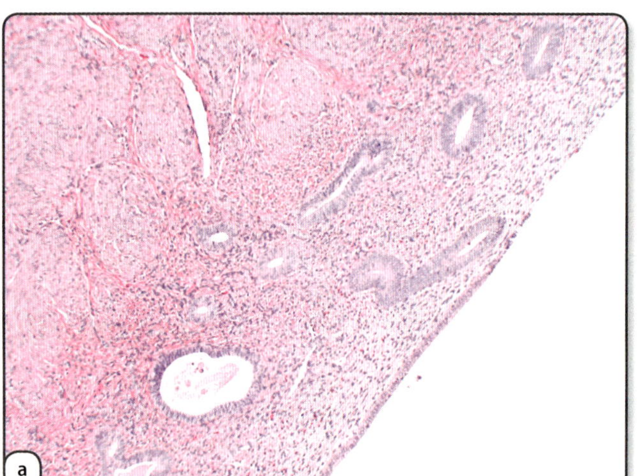

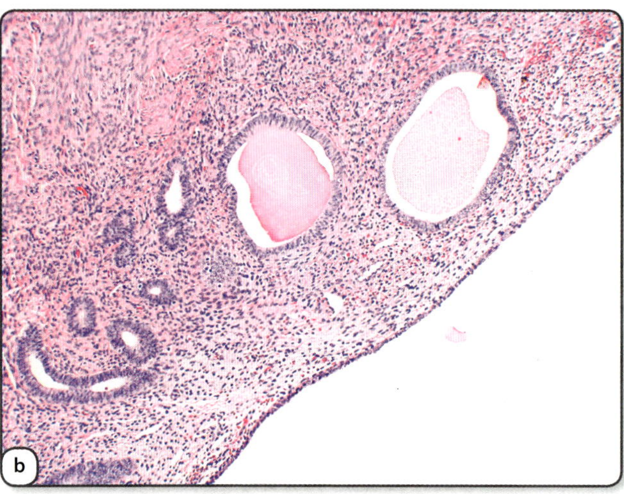

Figure 4.26 Atrophy. Note thinned endometrium (a). The endometrial glands show lack of mitotic activity, and have become smaller with less pseudostratification (b).

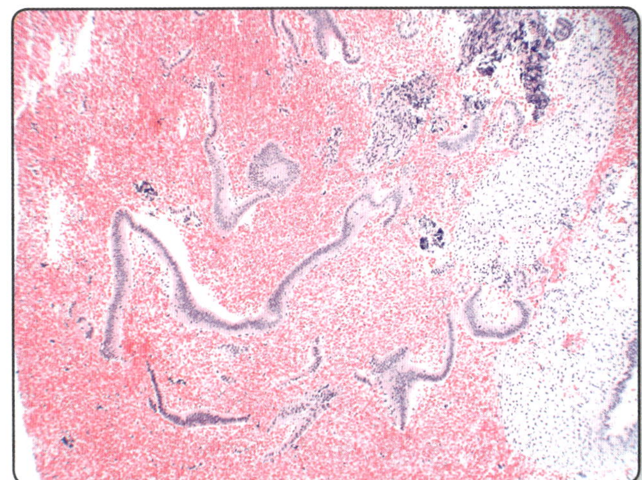

Figure 4.27 Atrophy. On biopsy, atrophy often appears as superficial strips of endometrium. While this finding is usually indicative of atrophy, other causes of scant tissue on biopsy must be considered.

References

1. Albers JR, Hull SK, Wesley RM. Abnormal uterine bleeding. Am Fam Physician. 2004;69:1915–26.
2. Lee SC, Kaunitz AM, Sanchez-Ramos L, Rhatigan RM. The oncogenic potential of endometrial polyps. A systemic review and meta-analysis. Obstet Gynecol 2010;116:1197–1205.
3. Heatley MK. Atypical polypoid adenomyoma: a systematic review of the English literature. Histopathology. 2006;48:609–10.
4. Ohishi Y, Kaku T, Kobayashi H, Aishima S, Umekita Y, Wake N, Tsuneyoshi M. CD10 immunostaining distinguishes atypical polypoid adenomyofibroma (atypical polypoid adenomyoma) from endometrial carcinoma invading the myometrium. Hum Pathol 2008;39:1446–53.
5. Smith M, Hagerty KA, Skipper B, Bocklage T. Chronic endometritis: a combined histopathologic and clinical review of cases from 2002 to 2007. Int J Gynecol Pathol 2009;29:44–50.
6. Pitsos M, Skurnick J, Heller DS. Chronic endometritis. The association of pathologic diagnoses with clinical findings J Reprod Med, 2009:54:373–77.
7. McCluggage WG. My approach to the interpretation of endometrial biopsies and curettings. J Clin Pathol 2006;59:801–12.
8. McCluggage WG. Miscellaneous disorders involving the endometrium. Semin Diagn Pathol 2010;27:287–310.
9. Boyle DP, McCluggage, WG. Combined actinomycotic and pseudoactinomycotic radiate granules in the female genital tract: description of a series of cases. J Clin Pathol 2009;62:1123–26.

5 Hormonally related abnormal uterine bleeding: dysfunctional uterine bleeding and exogenous hormone effects

Normal menstrual function is a delicate interplay of appropriate levels of estrogen and progesterone at appropriate times. When the balance is upset, abnormal bleeding patterns emerge, and this often leads to endometrial sampling. What complicates interpretation of these biopsies for the pathologist is the limited clinical history often accompanying the specimens. In addition, patients may have received exogenous hormones in an attempt to regulate their bleeding, and this history may not have been supplied. Exogenous hormonal effects may be superimposed on an underlying hyperplastic or neoplastic process, and this may present a confusing histologic picture. Communication between clinicians and pathologists will often help sort out confusing patterns, as well as lead to shorter, more useful reports, and is important for optimal patient care.

Dysfunctional uterine bleeding

In the absence of intrinsic uterine pathology, pregnancy-related issues, systemic disease, iatrogenic causes, hyperplasia or neoplasia, abnormal uterine bleeding can be attributed to dysfunctional uterine bleeding, which is secondary to hormonal imbalance. Most dysfunctional uterine bleeding (DUB) is anovulatory, and hence due to unopposed estrogen. However, ovulatory DUB can occur, and can manifest as a variety of secretory patterns. These may be in or out of phase, be weakly secretory, show gland/stromal dyssynchrony, or rarely present as irregular shedding or irregular ripening, discussed previously (**Figure 5.1**). More often, with anovulatory unopposed estrogenic stimulation, a variety of histopathological anovulatory patterns are seen. The endometrium may show atrophy or weakly proliferative changes (**Figure 5.2**), with less pseudostratification and no mitoses, or may simply show histologically normal proliferative features, with or without breakdown. The most common pattern is termed "disordered proliferation". The glands show proliferative features, with pseudostratification and mitotic activity. Occasionally dilated glands are seen, however there is no increase in the gland-to-stroma ratio, hence it is not hyperplastic

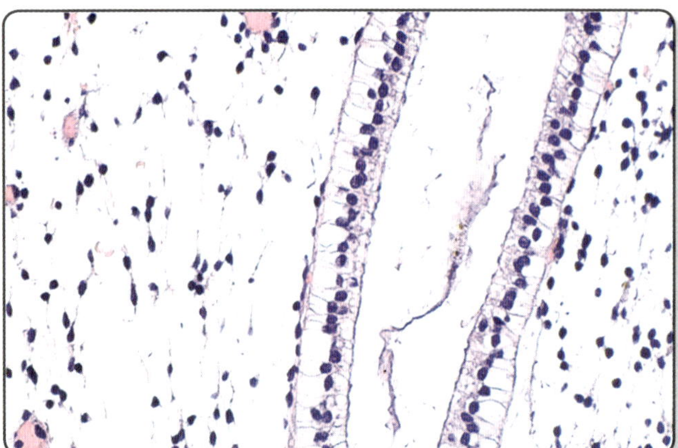

Figure 5.1 Dyssynchrony. The gland shows features of day 17, with stromal edema characteristic of day 22.

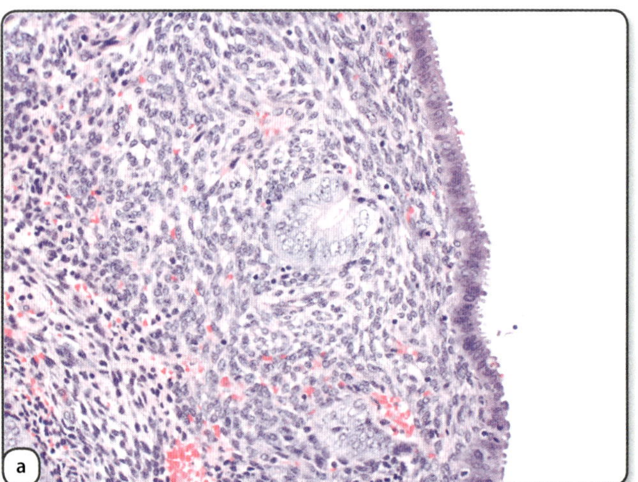

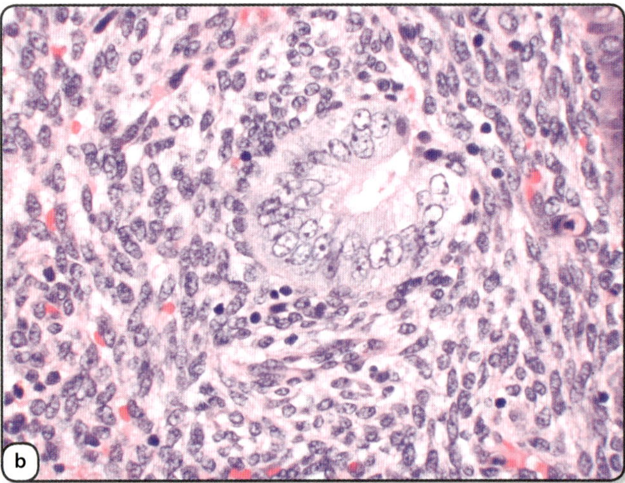

Figure 5.2 Weakly proliferative endometrium. The overall architecture of proliferative endometrium is maintained, however the glands are smaller, with less or no pseudostratification and no mitotic activity.

(**Figure 5.3**). Differences in the zonal distribution of calretinin have been demonstrated in women with dysfunctional uterine bleeding, both with and without histologic disordered proliferation, leading Mai et al[1] to the conclusion that there is an expansion of the stroma of the basalis into the functionalis. Superimposed exogenous or endogenous progesterone effect may present a confusing mix of findings (**Figure 5.4**).

In addition to the dysfunctional bleeding that may occur in women of reproductive age, the perimenopause is a time frequently marked by abnormal bleeding episodes, which may be due to the anovulation associated with ovarian senescence. Perimenopausal women often undergo endometrial biopsy, and a study by Boon et al of endometrial patterns in perimenopausal women, 41.5% showed abnormal secretory endometrium, 2% showed disordered proliferation, and 14.1% showed a mix of nonsecretory and secretory endometrium.[2]

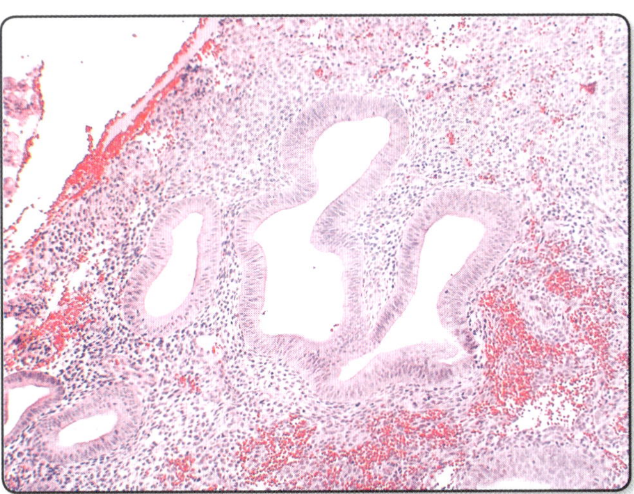

Figure 5.3 Disordered proliferation. Occasional glands are dilated, but there is no increase in gland-to-stromal ratio.

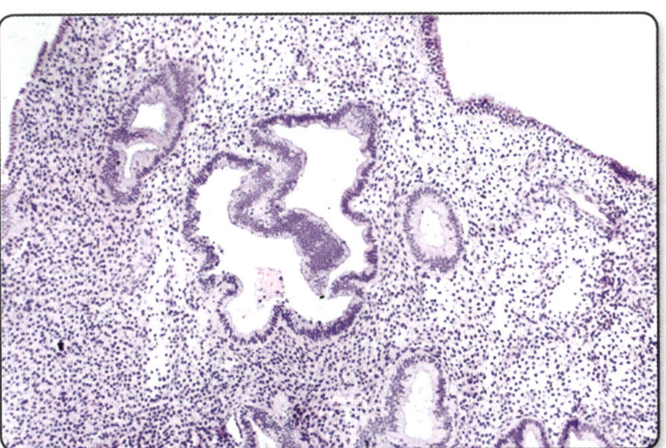

Figure 5.4 Disordered proliferation with superimposed secretory effect. Note the architecture of disordered proliferation with a few dilated glands, however glands show secretory features.

Exogenous hormonal causes of bleeding

Iatrogenic effects on the endometrium are often encountered by the pathologist. If a clinical history is provided, this may explain the histological features. There may be variability in the effects observed, depending on the drug, the dosage, the duration, and the underlying hormonal milieu of the patient. In addition, a clinical history of administration of exogenous hormones may not be provided. The approach to the "strange" biopsy is simple:

1. Is there enough tissue to make a diagnosis?
2. Is there any organic etiology for the bleeding?
3. Is there any evidence of hyperplasia or neoplasia?

In the absence of a specific diagnosis, and with an adequate specimen, a report of irregularly developed endometrium with no evidence of hyperplasia or neoplasia will usually serve the clinician who is providing care for the patient. Prolonged descriptions of the specific irregular features may be confusing.

Estrogen and hormone replacement therapy

The effects of unopposed estrogen on the endometrium are related to duration of exposure,[3] and can range from weakly proliferative to proliferative, through varying degrees of hyperplasia to frank carcinoma, usually of well-differentiated endometrioid histology. Hormone replacement therapy is a combination of estrogen and progesterone. The dosages and specific hormones utilized are different from oral contraceptives, and hence different patterns are seen. In addition, there are many different therapeutic regimens, and hence assigning a specific effect to a specific regimen is not practical. There may be either no change at all or a variety of mixed proliferative and secretory patterns, sometimes hyperplastic, sometimes with metaplastic changes as well. Breakdown may be seen.

If the history of hormonal therapy has been provided by the clinician, and there is no evidence of hyperplasia, a simple report may be provided, stating that there is benign but irregularly developed endometrium, consistent with hormone replacement therapy (HRT). In the absence a history of HRT, the pathologist is often left with providing a long descriptive diagnosis, as the patterns do not fit into any textbook category (**Figure 5.5**). Most significant pathology found on a biopsy of a woman on HRT reflects preexisting disease rather than disease secondary to the HRT.[4]

Progesterone

Progesterone therapy is often given to combat abnormal bleeding, and a history of exogenous progestins may not be provided to the pathologist. Although prolonged therapy with progestins may lead to atrophy, most often a distinct pattern is seen of pronounced decidualization of the endometrial stroma, with tiny inactive glands (**Figure 5.6**). Confusing

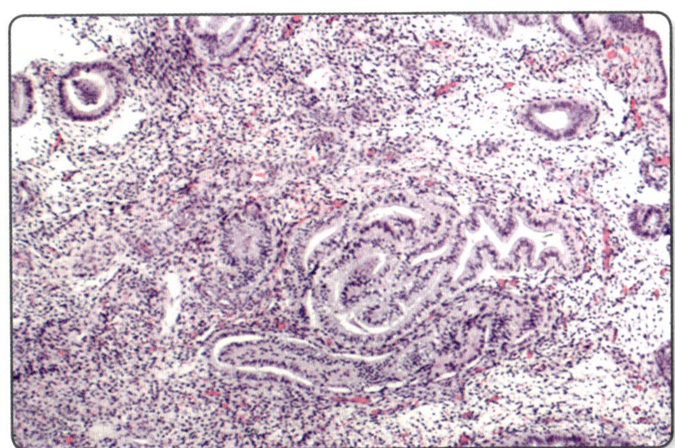

Figure 5.5 HRT. An irregular mixed pattern of proliferative and secretory features, with focal glandular crowding is seen.

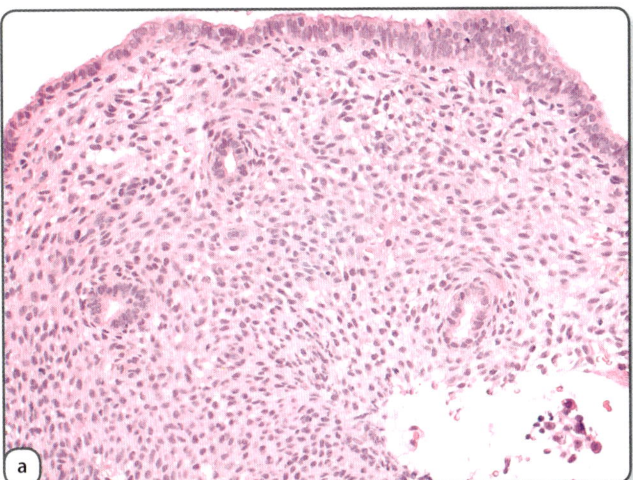

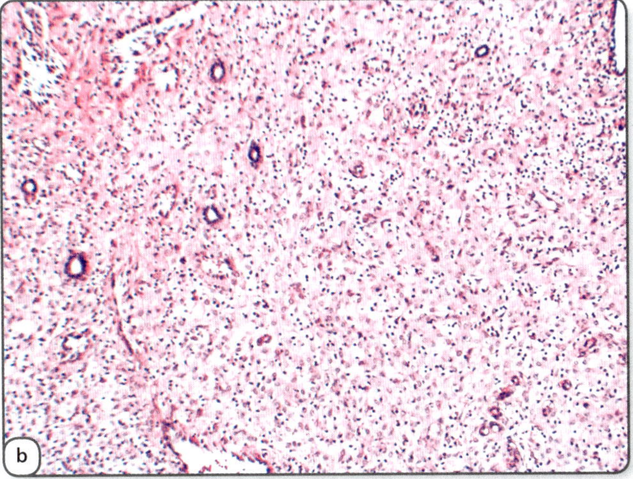

Figure 5.6 Progestin effect. The glands over time become small and inactive, with decidualization of the stroma (a). Note the tubal metaplasia on the surface. Over time, the decidualization becomes more pronounced, and the glands become tiny (b).

patterns emerge when the progesterone therapy is superimposed on an underlying hyperplasia or carcinoma, particularly in the absence of clinical history (**Figures 5.7–5.10**). The pathologist may be able to obtain the relevant history by communicating with the clinician, but may be left with providing a descriptive diagnosis.

Oral contraceptives

The progesterone effect of oral contraceptives predominates over the estrogenic effect.[3] Most oral contraceptives currently in use lead to an arrest of gland proliferation, stromal hyperplasia progressing to decidualization and eventual atrophy, and thin blood vessels. Initially, a dense spindled stroma may be seen (**Figure 5.11**), progressing through a phase indistinguishable from progestin therapy to, finally, atrophy.

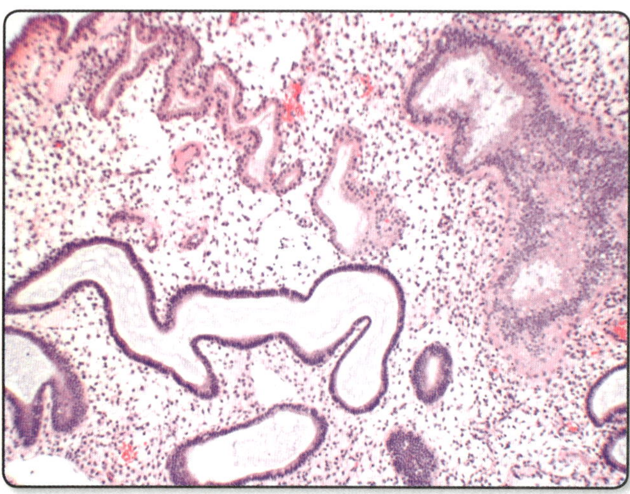

Figure 5.7 Presumed disordered proliferation with progestin effect, in the absence of clinical history. The architecture is consistent with disordered proliferation, however the cellular features suggest progestin effect.

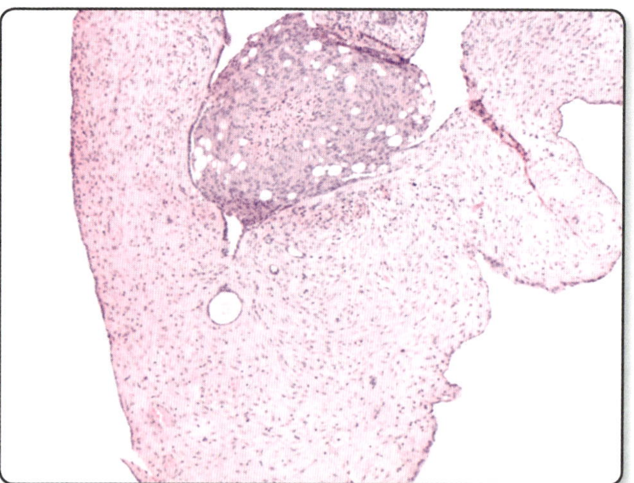

Figure 5.8 Progesterone effect on known simple hyperplasia. Note the characteristic glandular and stromal changes, with persistence of squamous metaplasia.

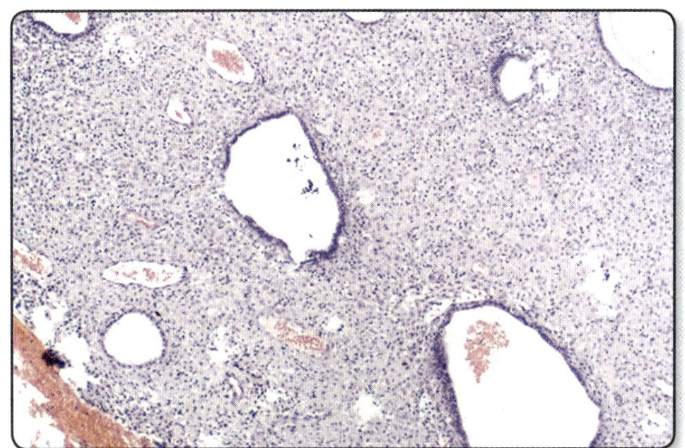

Figure 5.9 Progestin effect on simple hyperplasia. The dilated glands persist, however are no longer showing pseudostratification or mitoses. The stroma is decidualized.

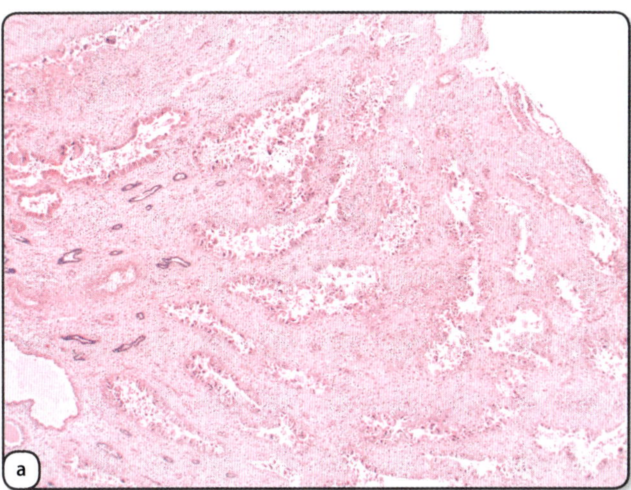

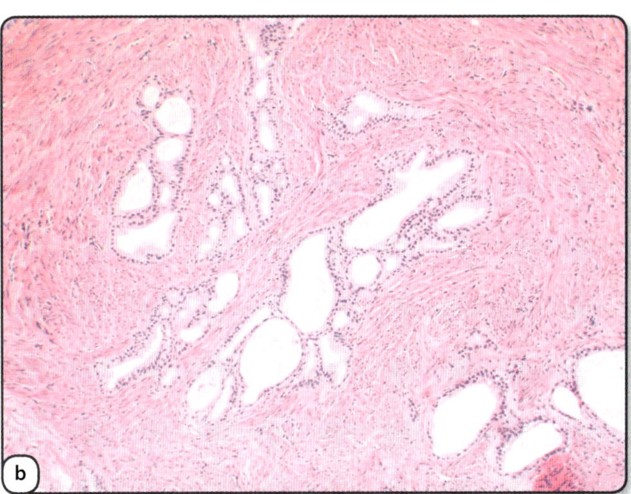

Figure 5.10 Uterine serous carcinoma with superimposed progestin effect (a). A combination of atrophic and neoplastic glands is seen in a decidualized stroma. Well differentiated endometrioid carcinoma invading myometrium (b), with superimposed secretory effect from a patient on megestrol acetate.

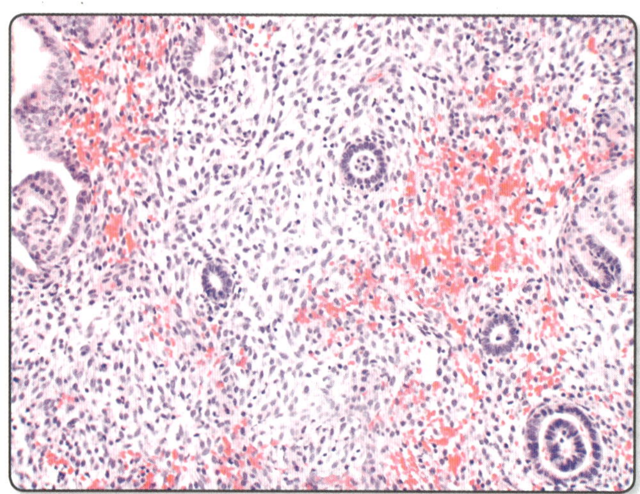

Figure 5.11 Oral contraceptive effects. Inactive glands in a spindle cell stroma.

Gonadotropin releasing hormone agonist (luprolide acetate)

Gonadotropin-releasing hormone agonist (leuprolide acetate) is utilized for its antiestrogenic activity, such as to shrink down leiomyomas before surgery, and to treat endometriosis. Endometrium from a treated patient becomes weakly proliferative, then inactive, and finally atrophic[3] (**Figure 5.12**). Amico et al described a case of a woman who underwent resectoscopic myomectomy after treatment with leuprolide acetate and was found to have diffuse squamous metaplasia of the endometrium.[5] The role of the leuprolide acetate is unclear here. The authors pointed out that a pitfall with this occurrence is the potential for misinterpretation of future curettings, when the squamous metaplasia could be mistaken for a carcinoma.

Ovulation induction drugs

Endometrial sampling used to be a part of the workup for infertility, although this is much less common now that serologic testing is

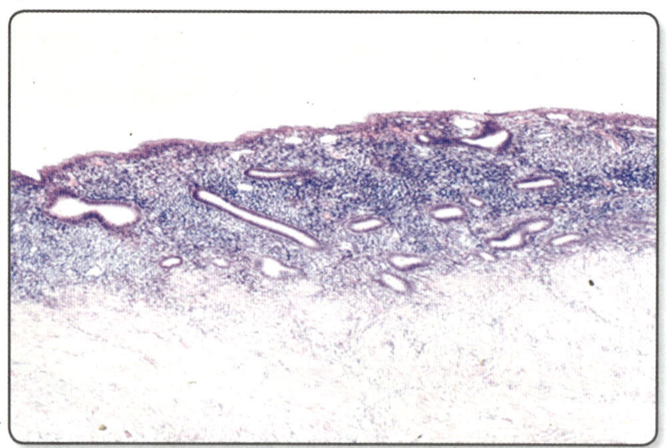

Figure 5.12 Leuprolide acetate. The endometrium has become atrophic.

available to assess ovulation. Rarely, pathology laboratories may receive endometrial samples from patients who have undergone ovulation induction therapy. Clomiphene citrate is associated with an exaggeration of the "piano-key" configuration seen on day 17 (**Figure 5.13**). The combination of Pergonal and hCG tends to produce dyssynchrony, with glandular features of day 17–18, and stromal features of day 22–23 (**Figure 5.14**).

Tamoxifen

Tamoxifen, used in breast cancer therapy, exerts an estrogenic effect on the postmenopausal endometrium. The most common pathology is endometrial polyps, more often developing malignancy than usual polyps[6] and often large, with a fibrous stroma[7,8] (**Figure 5.15**). Mucinous metaplasia may also be seen (**Figure 5.16**). Also occasionally associated are endometrial hyperplasia, carcinoma, and carcinosarcomas and sarcomas.[6] In one large series, about one-third of the patients had benign changes (polyps, hyperplasia, or metaplasia). Endometrial cancers were often high grade and invasive,[9] although the expected well-differentiated endometrioid carcinomas are also seen.

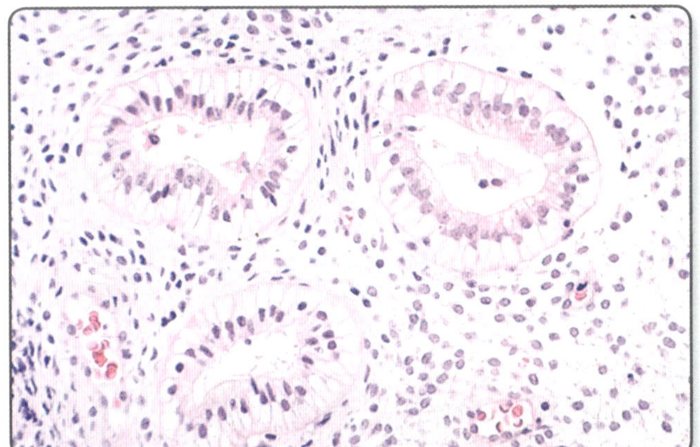

Figure 5.13 Clomiphene. Exaggerated day 17 glands are seen.

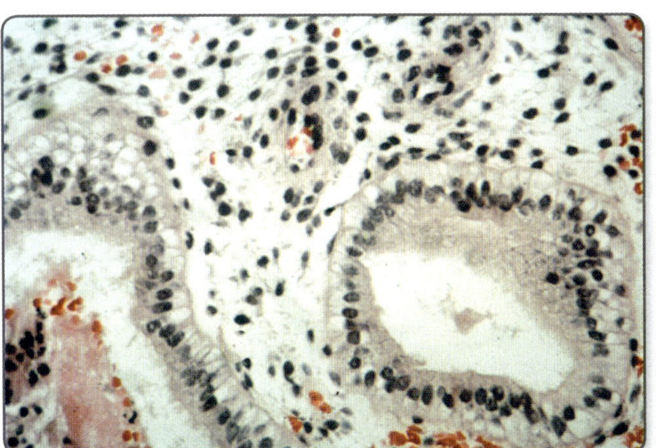

Figure 5.14 Pergonal/hCG. Dyssynchronous changes are seen, with day 17 glands, and day 22–23 stroma.

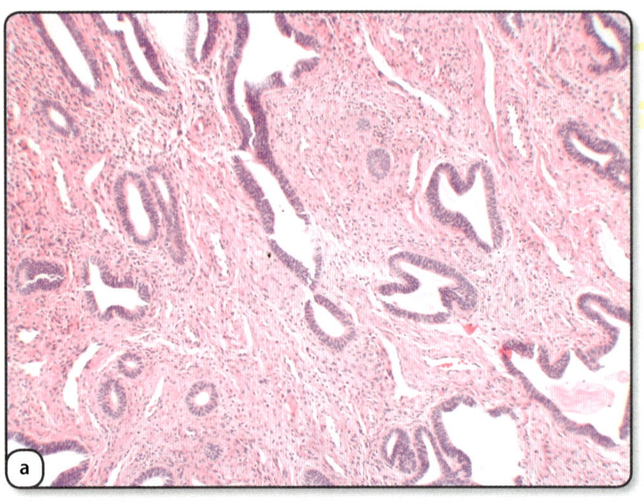

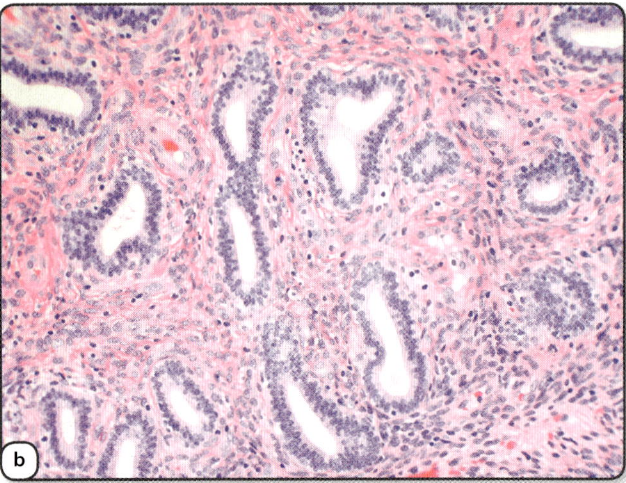

Figure 5.15 Tamoxifen. Polyps associated with tamoxifen are often quite large, with a dense fibrous stroma.

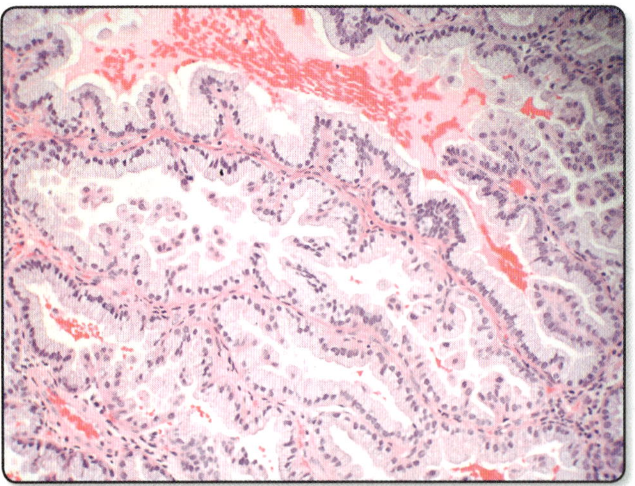

Figure 5.16 Tamoxifen. Mucinous metaplasia in a patient treated with tamoxifen.

Aromatase inhibitors

Patients switched to aromatase inhibitors from tamoxifen for their breast cancer treatment have been shown to experience less endometrial pathology, although it is unclear if the aromatase inhibitors are protective, or whether it is the cessation of tamoxifen that is providing the effect.[10]

Progesterone receptor modulators

Progesterone receptor modulators bind to endometrial progesterone receptors, and hence have a wide variety of potential therapeutic uses. They are used in the management of leiomyomata and endometriosis and in some cases as an abortifacient (mifepristone). The endometrial effects of progesterone receptor modulators have not been studied extensively, but they have been inconsistently found to show a unique pattern of asymmetric glandular stromal growth with cystically dilated glands showing mixed epithelium with estrogenic (mitotic) and progestational (secretory) features.[11] Fiscella et al described nonsynchronous endometrium, enlarged fluid filled glands, and abnormal blood vessels. The most common vascular change was thickwalled vessels, as seen in polyps, but some cases also showed capillary proliferation and dilated thin vessels in stroma.[12]

References

1. Mai KT, Teo I, Al Moghrabi H, Marginean Ec, Veinot JP. Calretinin and CD34 immunoreactivity of the endometrial stroma in normal endometrium and change of the immunoreactivity in dysfunctional uterine bleeding with evidence of "disordered endometrial stroma". Pathol 2008;40:493–99.
2. Boon J, Van de Putte SCJ, Scholten PC, Heintz APM. Histological patterns in endometrial samples from perimenopausal women. Maturitas 1999;32:155–59.
3. Deligdisch L. Hormonal pathology of the endometrium. Mod Pathol 2000;13: 285–94.
4. Feeley KM, Wells M. Hormone replacement therapy and the endometrium. J Clin Pathol 2001;54:435–40.
5. Amico P, Caltabiano R, Zizza G, Lanzafame S. About a case of diffuse endometrial squamous metaplasia after resectoscopic myomectomy: a potential diagnostic pitfall for gynecologists and pathologists. Appl Immunohistochem Mol Morphol 2010;18:392–95.
6. Cohen I. Endometrial pathologies associated with postmenopausal tamoxifen treatment. Gynecol Oncol 2004;94:256–66.
7. Varras M, Polyzos D, Akrivis Ch. Effects of tamoxifen on the human female genital tract: review of the literature. Eur J Gynaecol Oncol 2003;24:258–68.
8. Schlesinger C, Kamoi S, Ascher SM, Kendell M, Lage JM, Silverberg SG. Endometrial polyps: a comparison study of patients receiving tamoxifen with two control groups. Int J Gynecol Pathol 1998;17:302–11.
9. Deligdisch L, Kalir T, Cohen CJ, de Latour M, Le Bouedec G, Penault-Llorca. Endometrial histopathology in 700 patients treated with tamoxifen for breast cancer. Gynecol Oncol 2000;78:181–86.
10. Cohen I. Aromatase inhibitors and the endometrium. Maturitas 2008;59:285–92.
11. Mutter GL, Bergeron C, Deligdisch L, Ferenczy A, Glant M, Merino M et al. The spectrum of endometrial pathology induced by progesterone receptor modulators. Mod Pathol 2008;21:591–98.
12. Fiscella J, Bonfiglio T, Winters P, Eisinger SH, Fiscella K. Distinguishing features of endometrial pathology after exposure to the progesterone receptor modulator mifepristone. Hum Pathol 2011; 42: 947–53.

Simple hyperplasia without atypia (simple hyperplasia)

Simple hyperplasia is characterized by a mildly increased gland-to-stroma ratio. This is what distinguishes it from disordered proliferation, which also has occasionally cystic or outpouching glands but has no increase in gland-to-stroma ratio. In simple hyperplasia, the increased numbers of glands may show cystic dilatation or outpouchings ("rabbit ears"). The epithelium lining the glands is similar to that seen in proliferative endometrium, with oval nuclei without atypia. Mitotic activity is present (**Figures 6.1** and **6.2**).

A finding that should not be confused with simple hyperplasia is cystic atrophy (**Figure 6.3**). Cystic atrophy is a normal variant of atrophic endometrium, with flattened nonproliferating epithelium lining the cystic glands.

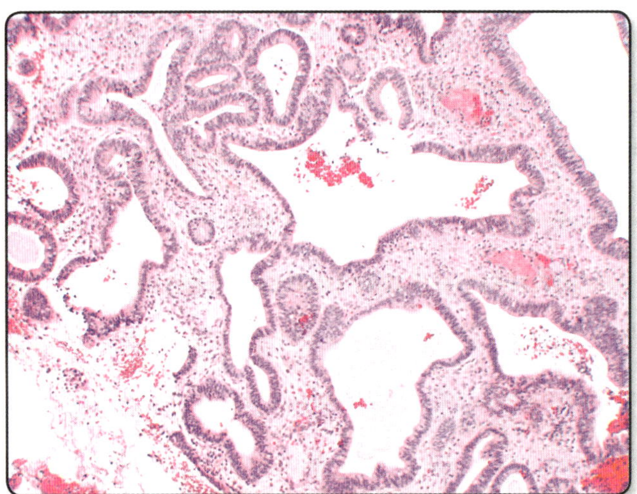

Figure 6.1 Simple hyperplasia, showing mild glandular crowding, with cystic dilatation and outpouchings of glands.

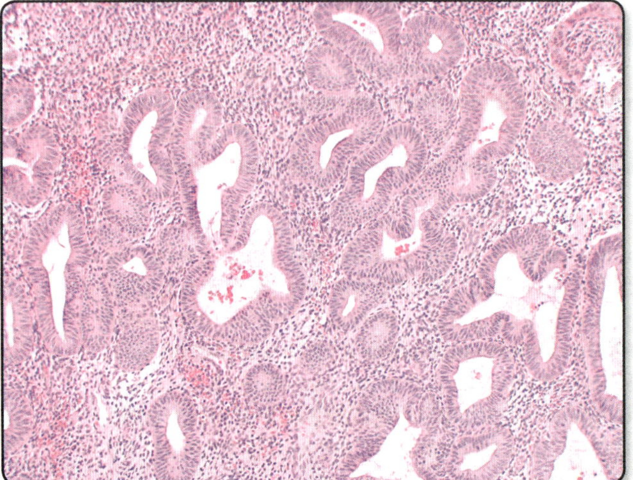

Figure 6.2 Simple hyperplasia. The epithelium is pseudostratified, with no nuclear atypia.

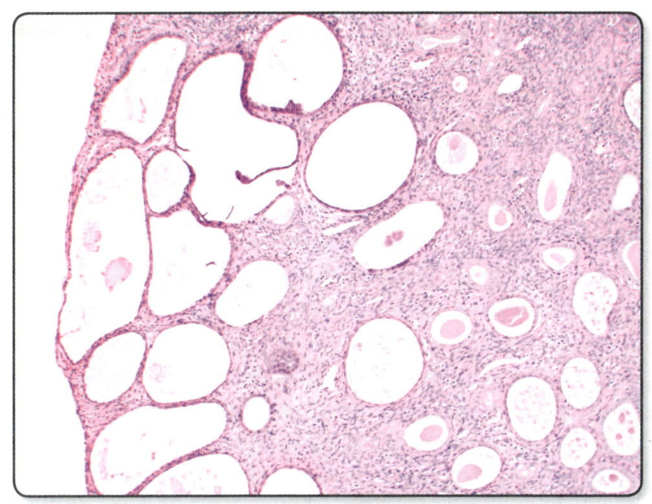

Figure 6.3 Cystic atrophy. Cystic glands show inactive epithelium.

Simple and other degrees of hyperplasia may also be noted within nests of adenomyosis, having no additional clinical significance beyond the diagnosis of hyperplasia of the lining (**Figure 6.4**).

The risk of simple hyperplasia progressing to carcinoma over 20 years in patients treated according to community standards was less than 5% in one study.[5] Simple hyperplasia is most often treated with progestational agents. Biopsies may be obtained as part of follow-up, and familiarity with superimposed progestational effect is important, particularly as a treatment history may not be provided (see p. 90).

Simple hyperplasia with atypia

Simple atypical hyperplasia is probably the least common pattern seen, and it is often not even mentioned in the classification, which is shortened to simple/complex/atypical. In simple hyperplasia with

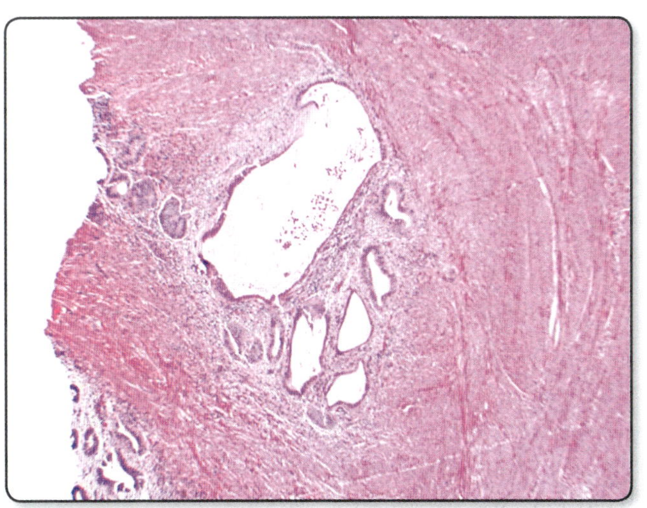

Figure 6.4 Simple hyperplasia within adenomyosis.

atypia, the architecture is the same as in simple nonatypical hyperplasia, but nuclear atypia is present. Atypical nuclei are enlarged and round rather than oval, with margination of the chromatin and clearing of the nucleus. Nucleoli may be seen. Nuclear pleomorphism and loss of polarity may be seen as well (**Figures 6.5** and **6.6**). Progression to carcinoma was seen in 8% (one patient) in the series reported by Kurman et al,[4] but this diagnosis occurs too uncommonly to conduct large studies.

Complex hyperplasia without atypia (complex hyperplasia)

Complex hyperplasia shows a greater degree of glandular crowding than simple hyperplasia (**Figures 6.7–6.10**). A range of changes may be seen in a single specimen, including areas of less crowding or simple hyperplasia, and accompanying metaplasias are often present. In the

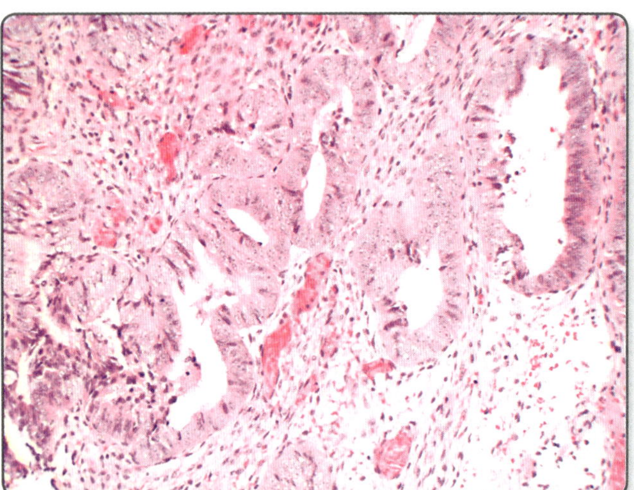

Figure 6.5 Simple hyperplasia with atypia. The architecture is only mildly crowded, but there is nuclear atypia.

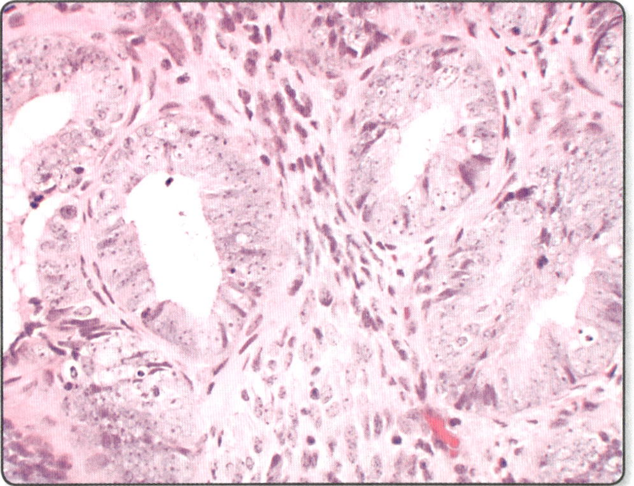

Figure 6.6 Simple hyperplasia with atypia. Nuclear atypia, with rounded nuclei, marginated chromatin with vesicular nuclei, with nucleoli seen.

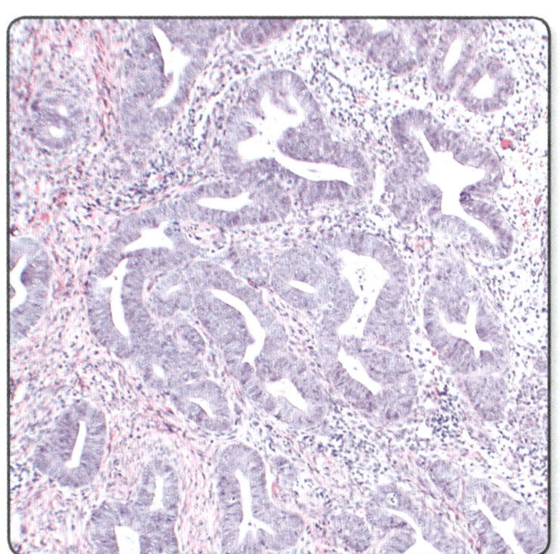

Figure 6.7 Complex hyperplasia showing increased gland-to-stromal ratio; however, stroma still intervenes.

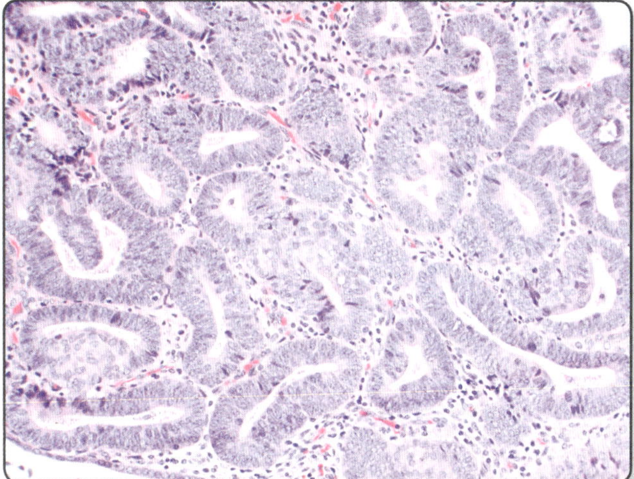

Figure 6.8 Complex hyperplasia showing increased gland-to-stromal ratio; however, stroma still intervenes.

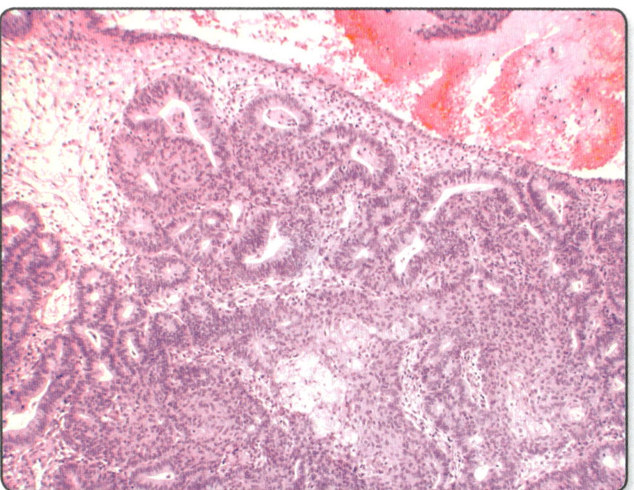

Figure 6.9 Complex hyperplasia with squamous metaplasia making the lesion appear more solid.

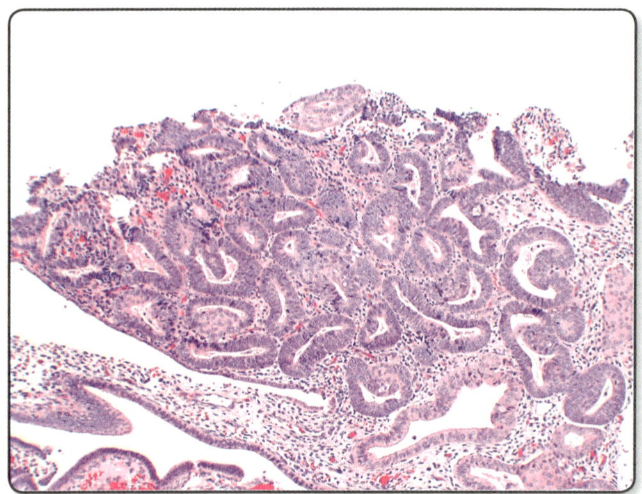

Figure 6.10 Range of types of hyperplasia, from simple on the bottom, to complex on the top. Squamous metaplasia is also seen.

absence of nuclear atypia, the risk of carcinoma is still low, with a 3% risk in the series reported by Kurman et al,[4] and less than 5% in the study by Lacey et al.[5]

The presence of squamous metaplasia may make the distinction of complex hyperplasia from well-differentiated adenocarcinoma difficult, particularly if there is minimal nuclear atypia in the carcinoma. Carcinoma by definition shows stromal invasion, as evidenced by stromal response, cribriforming, possible papillary configurations, and large masses of squamous epithelium. The last three criteria must be at least 2.1 mm in size, according to the criteria in the 1982 report by Kurman and Norris.[6] Often many fields have to be examined to make the distinction. Although the terminology is not in widespread use, Mittal et al have called lesions less than 2.1 mm but otherwise meeting the Kurman & Norris criteria as "adenocarcinoma in situ", and have found a greater likelihood of carcinoma and myometrial invasion by the carcinoma, in subsequent hysterectomies, after a biopsy diagnosis of adenocarcinoma in situ as they defined it.[7]

Atypical hyperplasia (complex hyperplasia with atypia)

Complex hyperplasia with atypia, or atypical hyperplasia, combines significant glandular crowding with nuclear atypia (**Figures 6.11–6.14**); although glands are crowded, some stroma remains. It may be difficult to distinguish from carcinoma if there is extensive squamous metaplasia.

Atypical hyperplasia has a high risk of either progression to carcinoma or concomitant carcinoma being present at hysterectomy after a diagnosis of atypical hyperplasia on biopsy. While most studies have estimated a risk of approximately 25%, one recent study estimated as high as 45.9%. [8] This being so, hysterectomy remains the treatment

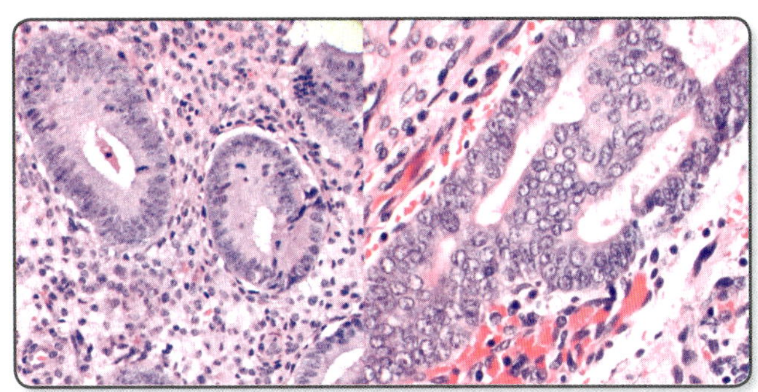

Figure 6.11 Nonatypical vs atypical nuclei. The nonatypical nuclei on the left are oval, with well-distributed chromatin. The larger rounder atypical nuclei on the right show vesiculation with margination of chromatin, loss of polarity, and occasional nucleoli.

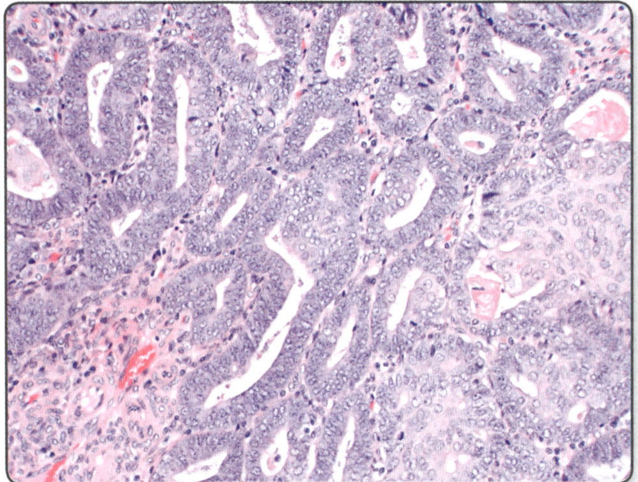

Figure 6.12 Atypical hyperplasia. Marked glandular crowding and nuclear atypia. Squamous metaplasia is also present.

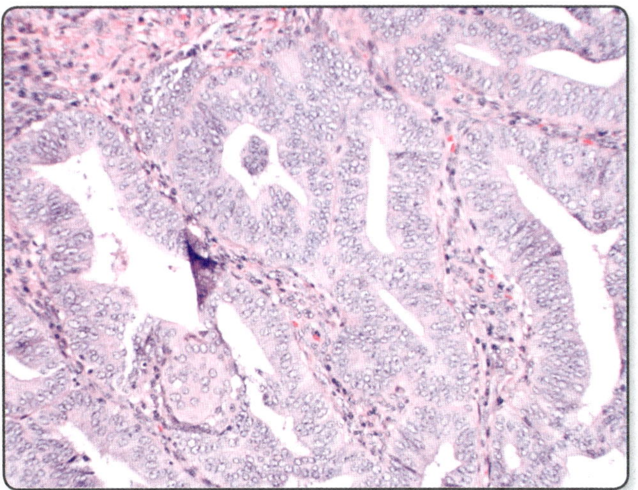

Figure 6.13 Atypical hyperplasia. Marked glandular crowding and nuclear atypia.

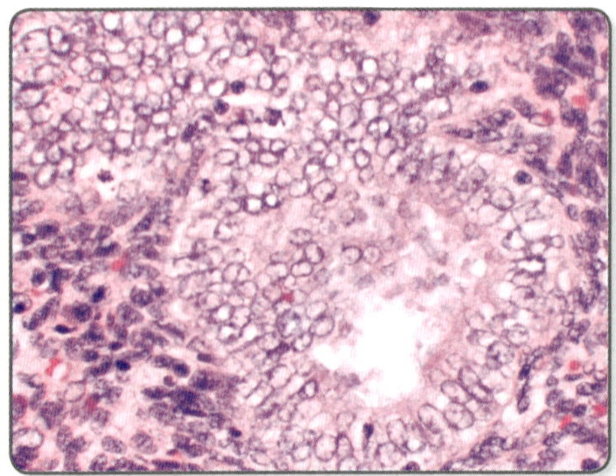

Figure 6.14 Atypical hyperplasia. Nuclei show marked vesiculation.

of choice for these lesions; however in extenuating circumstances, for example where medical therapy is chosen to preserve fertility, close follow-up is required. In a 20 year follow-up of patients, the risk associated with atypical hyperplasia progressing to carcinoma was one in eight at 10 years, and one in three at 20 years.[5]

EIN (endometrial intraepithelial neoplasia) terminology

The more recent EIN terminology was devised to incorporate genetic aspects of endometrial carcinogenesis as well as clinicopathologic aspects. While the original studies were performed morphometrically, the classification made available by Mutter and colleagues[3,11,13] for routine use is based on histology, and has been embraced by some as a more accurate way of predicting which lesions are at high risk of progressing to cancer.

While there does not seem to be major dispute that the WHO 94 classification is fraught with difficulty, the problem with the adoption of the EIN terminology on a widespread basis is concern that the original morphometric studies assigning risk do not reliably translate into day-to-day practice for the community pathologist. Most institutions would not find it practical to conduct morphometric diagnosis, due to cost and time restraints. There is also the issue of whether the H&E attempts at diagnosing EIN will be any more reproducible than WHO among working pathologists.[3,9] One study[10] suggested that in the hands of an experienced pathologist the WHO and EIN classifications have similar sensitivities and negative predictive values for coexistent endometrial cancer, but opined that the EIN system is more concrete, and hence may be preferable if an experienced pathologist is not available.[10] Sivridis et al[9] concluded that the EIN concept is impractical, but noted that both classifications focus on the recognition of cytologic atypia. Follow-up of at least 1 year in women with biopsy diagnosed atypical hyperplasia or EIN had similarly increased risks of progression to carcinoma in one study.[11] The debate continues, and at this juncture, both systems have their advocates.

In an attempt to educate pathologists on the use of the EIN system, Mutter and colleagues have set up a website with tutorials (www.endometrium.org). In an editorial on whether or not it is time to make the leap to this classification, Zaino has stated that this educational site is valuable in that in order to be useful, the terminology needs to be reproducible at the community pathologist level.[12] The terminology of the EIN classification is

- benign hyperplasia,
- EIN, and
- carcinoma.

Benign hyperplasia

Benign hyperplasia is defined as a polyclonal diffuse process which is hormonally dependent and not considered to be a significant risk for progressing to carcinoma.[3] It is thought of as a reactive process amenable to hormonal therapy.

EIN

EIN is a monoclonal proliferation, initially localized, which can progress to a more diffuse distribution. It is a neoplastic proliferation.[3] The morphologic correlate of the morphometric EIN (based on a D-score) is defined predominantly by the volume percent stroma (VPS). Lesions with less than 55% VPS are often monoclonal and thus may represent EIN, while lesions with over 55% VPS are usually polyclonal[3] and hence represent endometrial hyperplasia. While phosphatase and tensin homolog (PTEN) inactivation (and immunonegativity), is the molecular pathway of endometrioid carcinoma, and is seen in two-thirds of cases of EIN, it often precedes any recognizable histologic changes, and is often focally present in normal endometrium, as well as being present in some EIN cases, making it a very nonspecific test.[3] The other criteria for the histologic diagnosis of EIN besides VPS less than 55% are that in the same lesional area the cytology of the crowded focus differs from the background, the maximum linear aspect of the lesion exceeds 1 mm, and benign mimics and cancer have been ruled out.[3] Applying EIN criteria was felt to outperform the WHO classification, and it showed good interobserver agreement between three gynecologic pathologists in one study.[13] EIN is thought to be best treated with hysterectomy, however hormonal therapy with follow-up is an option (**Figure 6.15**).

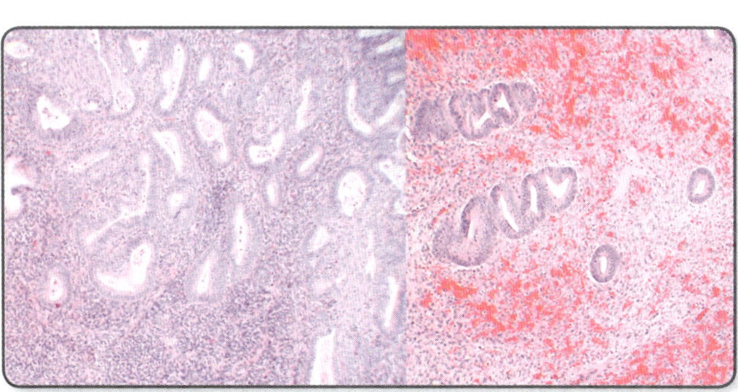

Figure 6.15 Intraepithelial neoplasia (EIN). Both fields are from the same biopsy. The focus of EIN on the left was present in a biopsy dominated by the proliferative endometrium on the right.

Precursors of type 2 uterine serous carcinoma

Endometrial intraepithelial carcinoma (EIC)

EIC had originally been thought to be the precursor lesion of serous adenocarcinoma of the endometrium, often seen in association with invasive serous carcinoma.[14] However, more recently some authors have stated that EIC actually represents early serous carcinoma, since it doesn't behave as a precancer. EIC is defined as cells identical to serous carcinoma, arising on the surface of the endometrium and devoid of stromal or myometrial invasion (**Figure 6.16a**). However, as extrauterine disease is the major prognostic factor for these early lesions, and disseminated disease has been found with EIC, Wheeler et al now call EIC "minimal uterine serous carcinoma" and combine it with serous carcinomas measuring ≤ 1 cm.[15]

Proposed as a better candidate precursor lesion for serous carcinoma is an entity called "endometrial glandular dysplasia",[16] which shows a p53 staining pattern and Ki-67 index intermediate between normal endometrium (p53 negative and Ki-67 low) and EIC (p53 staining strong and diffusely present, and Ki-67 index elevated), and has a lesser degree of nuclear atypia.[17] It is a surface lesion, often only occupying a gland or two, and it may have some papillary or cribriform architecture, and some nuclear atypia with loss of polarity and presence of nucleoli, but less than EIC. As such, this may be a difficult lesion to diagnose (**Figure 6.16b** and **c**). This lesion has been found in retrospective biopsy material from serous carcinomas, consistent with a precursor lesion.[18]

Superimposed therapeutic effects on endometrial hyperplasia

Secretory hyperplasia, the presence of secretory glands in a crowded configuration with markedly increased gland-to-stromal ratio, is thought to be a transient progestational effect on hyperplasia, either endogenously from ovulation, or exogenously (**Figure 6.17**)

Progestin effect on hyperplasia may show the remnants of the architecture, with inactive or secretory glands in a decidualized stroma (**Figure 6.18**). In a study of treated atypical hyperplasia and well-differentiated carcinoma, Wheeler et al[19] noted decrease in the gland-to-stroma ratio, decreased or absent mitotic activity, and loss of atypia, and they confirmed that the architectural abnormalities persisted longer. Eosinophilic, secretory, squamous, and mucinous metaplasia were seen after therapy. In some cases, treatment induced papillary or cribriform architecture, mimicking progression.

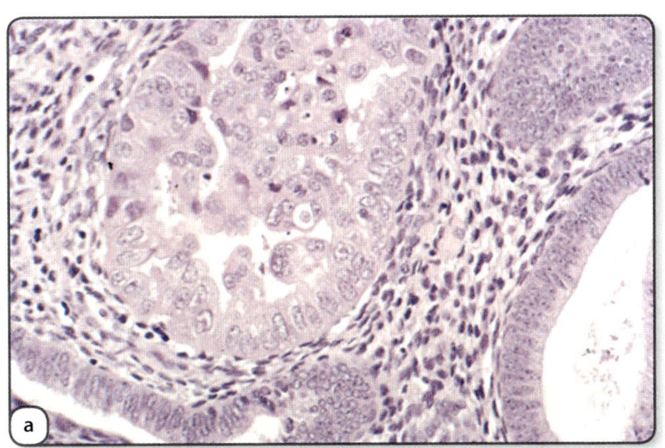

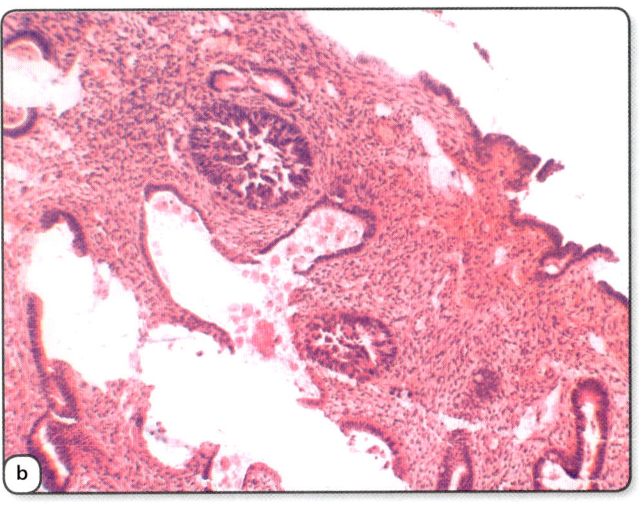

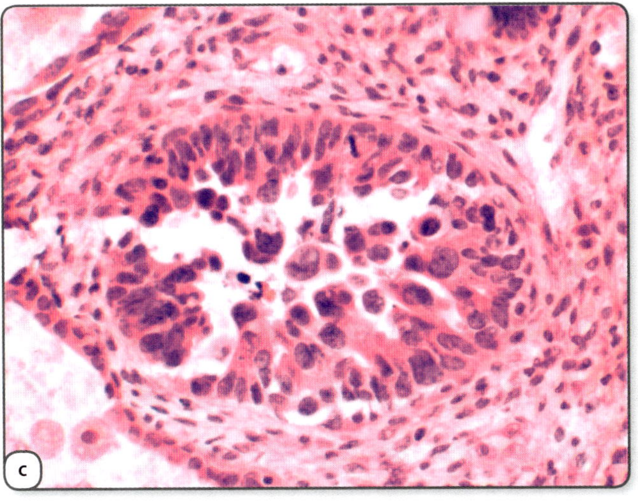

Figure 6.16 Endometrial intraepithelial carcinoma showing marked cytologic atypia. (a) Endometrial glandular dysplasia showing single dysplastic glands. (b) Admixed with nondysplastic glands, with cytologic atypia less than seen in EIC (c).

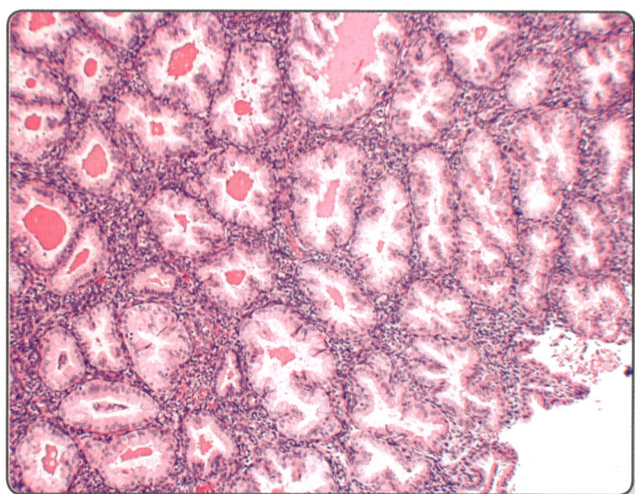

Figure 6.17 Secretory hyperplasia. There is marked crowding of secretory glands

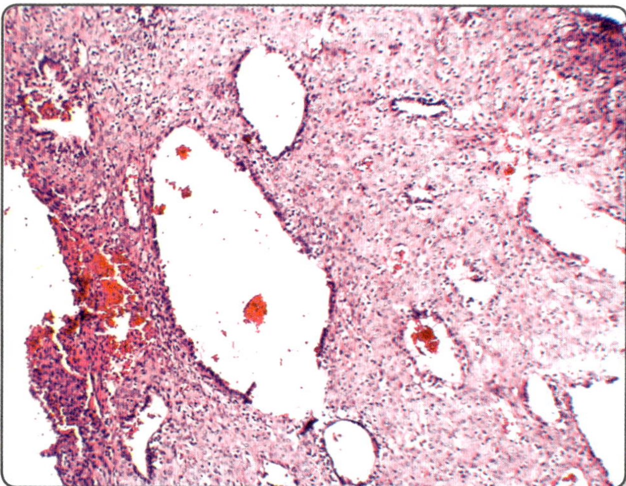

Figure 6.18 Simple hyperplasia after progesterone therapy, showing preservation of the architectural abnormality in a decidualized stroma.

References

1. Allison KH, Reed SD, Voigt LF, Jordan CD, Newton KM, Garcia RL. Diagnosing endometrial hyperplasia: why is it so difficult to agree? Am J Surg Pathol 2008;32:691–98.
2. Sherman ME, Ronnett BM, Ioffe OB, Richesson DA, Rush BB, et al. Reproducibility of biopsy diagnoses of endometrial hyperplasia: evidence supporting a simplified classification. Int J Gynecol Pathol 2008;27:318–25.
3. Baak JP, Mutter GL. EIN and WHO94. J Clin Pathol 2005;58:1–6.
4. Kurman RJ, Kaminski PF, Norris HJ. The behavior of endometrial hyperplasia. A long-term study of "untreated" hyperplasia in 170 patients. Cancer 1985;56:403–12.
5. Lacey JV Jr, Sherman ME, Rush BB, Ronnett BM, Ioffe OB, Duggan MA, et. al. Absolute risk of endometrial carcinoma during 20-year follow-up among women with endometrial hyperplasia. J Clin Oncol 2010;28: 788–92.
6. Kurman RJ, Norris HJ. Evaluation of criteria for distinguishing atypical endometrial hyperplasia from well-differentiated carcinoma. Cancer 1982;49:2547–59.

7. Mittal K, Sebenik M, Irwin C, Yan Z, Popiolek D, et al. Presence of endometrial adenocarcinoma in situ in complex atypical endometrial hyperplasia is associated with increased incidence of endometrial carcinoma in subsequent hysterectomy. Mod Pathol 2009;22:37–42.
8. Pennant S, Manek S, Kehoe S. Endometrial atypical hyperplasia and subsequent diagnosis of endometrial cancer: a retrospective audit and literature review. J Obstet Gynaecol 2008;28:632–33.
9. Sivridis E, Giatromanolaki A. The endometrial hyperplasias revisited. Virchows Arch 2008;453:223–31.
10. Salman MC, Usubutun A, Boynukalin K, Yuce K. Comparison of WHO and endometrial intraepithelial neoplasia classifications in predicting the presence of coexistent malignancy in endometrial hyperplasia. J Gynecol Oncol 2010;21:97–101.
11. Lacey JV, Mutter GL, Nucci MR, Ronnett BM, Ioffe OB, et al. Risk of subsequent endometrial carcinoma associated with endometrial intraepithelial neoplasia (EIN) classification of endometrial biopsies. Cancer 2008;113:2073–81.
12. Zaino RJ. Endometrial hyperplasia: is it time for a quantum leap to a new classification? Int J Gynecol Pathol 2000;19:314–21.
13. Hecht JL, Ince TA, Baak JPA, Baker HE, Ogden MW, Mutter GL. Prediction of endometrial carcinoma by subjective EIN diagnosis. Mod Pathol 2005;18:324–30.
14. Ambros RA, Sherman ME, Zahn CM, Bitterman P, Kurman RJ. Endometrial intraepithelial carcinoma: a distinctive lesion specifically associated with tumors displaying serous differentiation. Hum Pathol 1995;26:1260–67.
15. Wheeler DT, Bell KA, Kurman RJ, Sherman ME. Minimal uterine serous carcinoma: diagnosis and clinicopathologic correlation. Am J Surg Pathol 2000;24:797–806.
16. Zheng W, Liang SX, Yu H, Rutherford T, Chambers SK, Schwartz PE. Endometrial glandular dysplasia: a newly defined precursor lesion of uterine papillary serous carcinoma. Part I: morphologic features. Int J Surg Pathol 2004;12:207–23.
17. Yi X, Zheng W. Endometrial glandular dysplasia and endometrial intraepithelial neoplasia.Curr Opin Obstet Gynecol 2008;20:20–25.
18. Zheng W, Liang SX, Yi X, Ulukus EC, Davis JR, Chambers SK. Occurrence of endometrial glandular dysplasia precedes uterine papillary serous carcinoma. Int J Gynecol Pathol 2007;26:38–52.
19. Wheeler T, Bristow RE, Kurman RJ. Histologic alterations in endometrial hyperplasia and well-differentiated carcinoma treated with progestins. Am J Surg Pathol 2007;31:988–98.

7 Endometrial malignancies

Endometrial malignancies are histologically classified according to the World Health Organization (WHO) classification[1] (**Table 7.1**). As more is learned about the molecular and genetic mechanisms of endometrial malignancies and their impact on prognosis, the classification of and treatment planning for endometrial malignancies are evolving. This chapter reviews the histopathology of endometrial malignancies (for discussion of updates in our understanding of molecular mechanisms, see Chapter 9).

Biologic and molecular classification

Endometrial carcinomas have been divided into those that are estrogen related, and those that are not estrogen related.[2] The estrogen-related type 1 tumors include endometrioid adenocarcinoma and variants, while those unrelated to estrogen, the type 2 tumors, are predominantly composed of serous and (less often) clear cell adenocarcinomas. The patient demographics are different: type 1 patients are more likely to be younger postmenopausal women, heavier, and Caucasian; type 2 cancers are disproportionally represented in more elderly thinner African-American women.[3–5] Prognoses differ significantly, with overall 5-year survival about 74% for type 1 and 27–42% for type 2.[6] Risk factors for type 1 are primarily related to hyperestrogenism, and include earlier menarche/later menopause, unopposed exogenous estrogen or endogenous estrogen (i.e. from polycystic ovarian disease or an estrogen-secreting ovarian tumor), diabetes, hypertension, tamoxifen therapy, as well as Lynch syndrome (hereditary nonpolyposis coli colorectal cancer). The risk factors for type 2 cancers are less well elucidated. Type 1 and type 2 cancers have different molecular pathways, which will be discussed in detail in Chapter 9.

Histopathologic classification of endometrial carcinoma

Endometrioid adenocarcinoma

Endometrial cancer is the fourth most common cancer in women in the USA,[7] and the most common gynecologic cancer in Western Europe and North America.[8] It is more common in North America and Europe than in Africa and Asia.[6] Endometrioid adenocarcinoma represents about

WHO classification of endometrial neoplasms		
Epithelial tumors	Endometrial carcinoma	• Endometrioid adenocarcinoma and variants (squamous differentiation, villoglandular, secretory, ciliated cell) • Mucinous adenocarcinoma • Serous adenocarcinoma • Clear cell adenocarcinoma • Mixed cell adenocarcinoma • Squamous cell carcinoma • Transitional cel l carcinoma • Small cell carcinoma • Undifferentiated carcinoma • Other
	Endometrial hyperplasia	See Chapter 6†
Mesenchymal tumors	Endometrial stromal and related tumors	• Endometrial stromal nodule • Endometrial stromal sarcoma, low-grade • Undifferentiated endometrial sarcoma
	Smooth muscle tumors†	
	Miscellaneous mesenchymal tumors†	
Mixed epithelial mesenchymal tumors		• Carcinosarcoma (malignant mixed Müllerian tumor) • Adenosarcoma • Carcinofibroma • Adenofibroma • Adenomyoma • Atypical polypoid variant
Gestational trophoblastic disease		See Chapter 3†
Miscellaneous tumors†		
Lymphoid and haematopoietic tumors†		
Secondary tumors†		

† Details of table confined to the discussed entities. See Tavassoli and Devilee[1] for further details on the other entities.

Table 7.1 WHO classification of endometrial neoplasms. Adapted from Tavassoli and Devilee.[1]

80% of endometrial cancers.[9] Clinically, the most common presentation is post-menopausal bleeding, defined as any bleeding occurring after a year of amenorrhea. Although most cases of postmenopausal bleeding are related to atrophy, all cases must be investigated.

Grossly, endometrial cancer may be focal or diffuse. Uteri are often submitted for intraoperative consul tation to assess the depth of invasion. Although this can often be ascertained grossly, particularly if there is an advancing tumor front rather than individual gland invasion, it may not be possible to accurately assess it until microscopy is available. Leiomyomata may further obscure a gross assessment.

Microscopically, the appearance of the tumor varies greatly by grade. Unlike many other neoplasms, where grading is based on degree of cytologic atypia, in endometrioid adenocarcinoma, the grading is based predominantly on percentage of solid versus glandular tumor, not counting solid areas due to squamous differentiation. A well-differentiated FIGO grade 1 tumor is no more than 5% solid, FIGO grade 2 (moderately differentiated) is 6–50% solid, and anything over 50% solid is a grade 3 (poorly differentiated) tumor (**Figures 7.1–7.3**). The glandular epithelium shows only minimal atypia in most cases, resembling proliferative glands, and significant and diffuse nuclear atypia allows upgrading by one grade. Grading of endometrial adenocarcinoma can be problematic with poor reproducibility.[10] It has been shown that there is often a discrepancy between the grade on endometrial curettage and subsequent hysterectomy, due to sampling variation.[11] Some authors[10,12] have suggested a binary system of grading, feeling that hematoxylin and eosin (H&E) microscopy can only

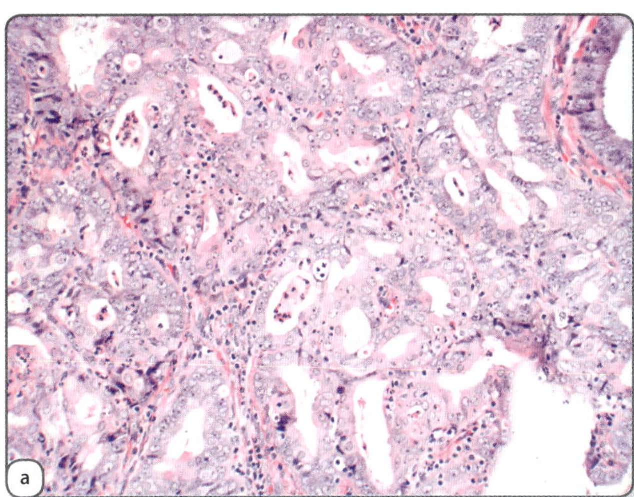

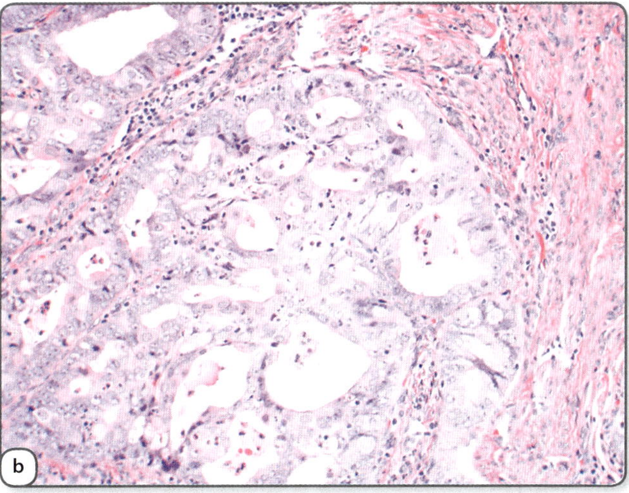

Figure 7.1 Well differentiated (FIGO grade 1) endometrial adenocarcinoma, endometrioid type, showing back-to-back glands (a), and cribriforming (b).

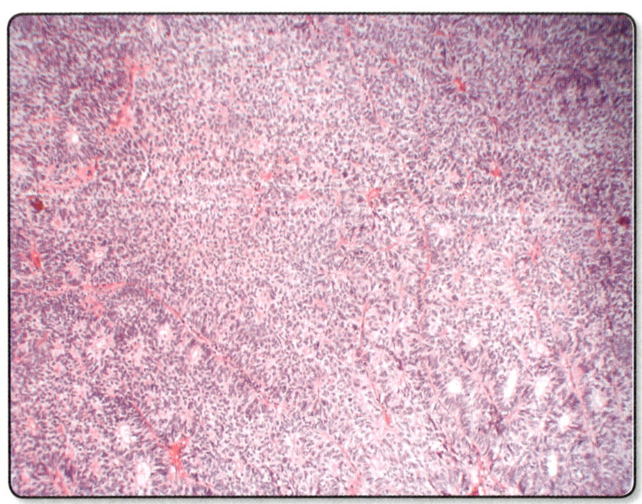

Figure 7.2 Moderately differentiated (FIGO grade 2) endometrial adenocarcinoma, endometrioid type. Note glandular area on right, and more solid area on left.

distinguish low and high grade, and that any further prognostication probably will require molecular markers in the future.

Microscopically, in the glandular portions of the tumor, there is lack of endometrial stroma, with back-to-back glands, sometimes with cribriforming ("gland within gland"). This lack of endometrial stroma is what makes the lesion an invasive carcinoma. Desmoplastic reaction is rare in the absence of myometrial invasion. Adjacent hyperplasia is present in up to 45% of cases.[9] In curettage specimens, the presence of pyometra (**Figure 7.4**) is a sign that endometrial carcinoma may be present, and probably occurs in association with tumor necrosis and cervical canal obstruction. If pyometra is present without carcinoma on curettage, clinical correlation is advised, as a cancer may not have been sampled. At hysterectomy, it is possible that a tumor may have been removed at curettage, and therefore there may be no residual tumor found, particularly if the lesion was focal.

The final reported depth of invasion is assessed microscopically and contributes to tumor staging. Depth is measured from the endometrial/myometrial interface to the deepest point of myometrial invasion, as a percentage of myometrial thickness (**Figure 7.5**). This endometrial/myometrial interface may be difficult to evaluate, as normal endometrium may not be present on the same slide as the deepest tumor, but can be approximated from a different section. If the myometrial wall is thick, the full thickness of the uterus can be placed in two paired and so designated tissue cassettes to assess the measurement. In a review of cases, Ali et al[13] acknowledged the difficulty in this area, particularly in cases of exophytic tumors, irregular endomyometrial junctions, adenomyosis, and extensive stromal smooth muscle metaplasia.

The most recent FIGO staging is based on a furthering of our knowledge of prognosis since the previous version in 1988. It now

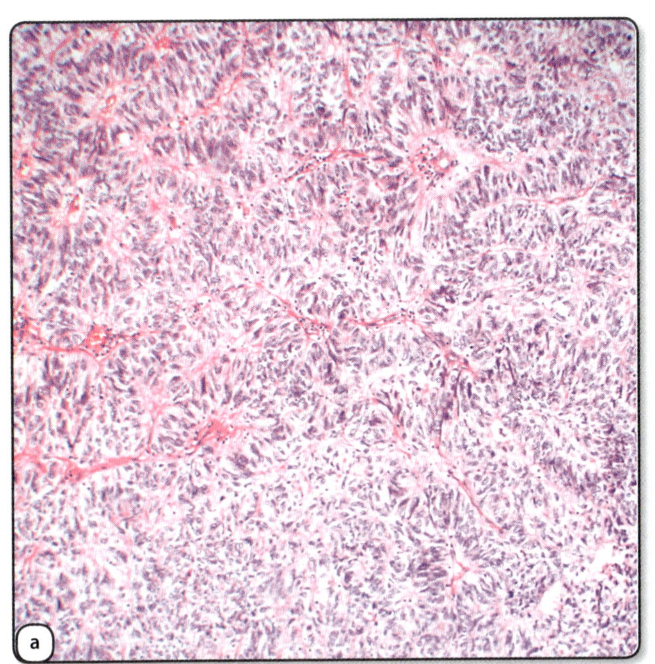

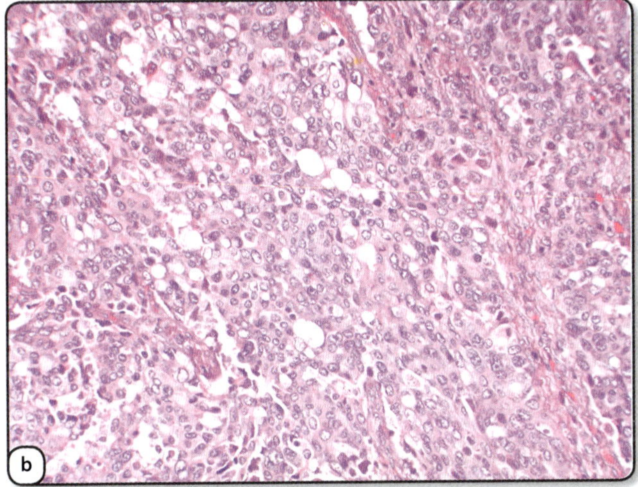

Figure 7.3 Poorly differentiated (FIGO grade 3) endometrial adenocarcinoma, endometrioid type. Although solid, overall the glandular nature sometimes more easily appreciated (a) than in other cases (b).

divides tumor depth into IA (less than one-half), and IB (one-half or greater), combining the older IA and IB into IA. In this new staging, only cervical stromal, not glandular, involvement upstages to a stage II, and pelvic and para-aortic nodal involvement have been separated[14,15] (**Table 7.2**). The staging applies to all grades of tumor. Notations include that endocervical glandular involvement without cervical involvement remains a stage I, and that positive cytology does not change the stage but needs to be separately reported.

A potentially problematic area is the involvement of adenomyotic foci by carcinoma, since this is not thought to alter prognosis in the way

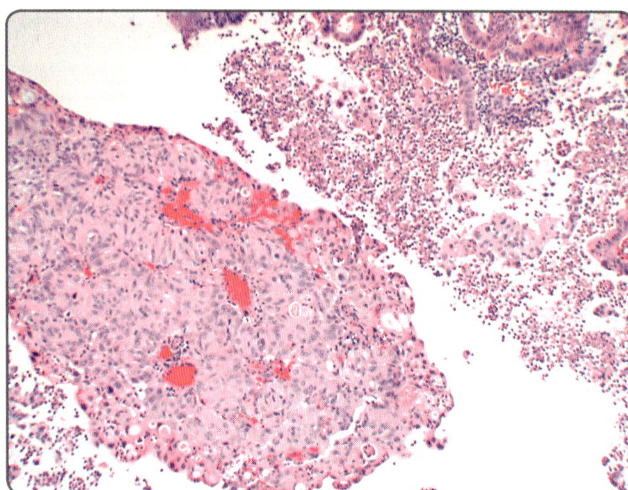

Figure 7.4 Endometrial adenocarcinoma in a curettage, in a background of pyometra.

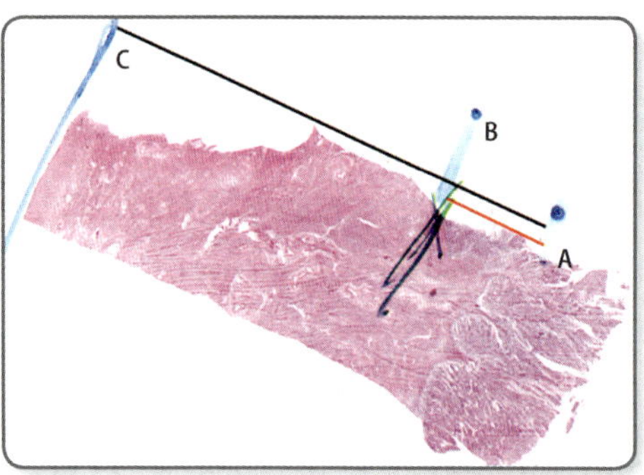

Figure 7.5 Depth of invasion measured from the normal endometrial/myometrial interface, to the deepest portion of invasion, and expressed as the percent myometrial invasion. In this case it is 5 mm (from A to B) out of 23 mm (A to C), or 22%.

that myometrial invasion does.[9,16] Helpful hints include the presence of non-neoplastic adenomyosis in the uterus and in the foci in question, the presence of endometrial stroma, and/or benign endometrial glands. CD10 will stain endometrial stroma; however, it will also stain the cells immediately around glands invading myometrium, so its usefulness is limited, although negative CD 10 will rule out adenomyosis.[17] It has also been pointed out that the finding of carcinoma in adenomyosis at the time of frozen section needs to be recognized, avoiding the pitfall of diagnosing excessively deep invasion.[18] Other potential mimics of endometrioid carcinoma include artifactual papillarity of glands, squeeze artifact (or telescoping), menstrual collapse mimicking glandular crowding (this is usually seen on curettage), intravascular menstrual endometrium, adenomyosis with atrophic stroma, intravascular adenomyosis, squamous metaplasia, atypical polypoid adenomyoma, and radiation atypia.[9]

There is still debate on whether pelvic lymph node dissection is of any benefit in early-stage cancer. Approximately 10% of women with stage I carcinomas will have nodal involvement.[8] There have been a few studies on sentinel node biopsies, however the identification rate for

FIGO staging of carcinoma of the endometrium	
Stage I*	Tumor confined to the corpus uteri
IA*	No or less than half myometrial invasion
IB*	Invasion equal to or more than half of the myometrium
Stage II*	Tumor invades cervical stroma, but does not extend beyond the uterus**
Stage III*	Local and/or regional spread of the tumor
IIIA*	Tumor invades the serosa of the corpus uteri and/or adnexae†
IIIB*	Vaginal and/or parametrial involvement†
IIIC*	Metastases to pelvic and/or para-aortic lymph nodes†
IIIC1*	Positive pelvic nodes
IIIC2*	Positive para-aortic lymph nodes with or without positive pelvic lymph nodes
Stage IV*	Tumor invades bladder and/or bowel mucosa, and/or distant metastases
IVA*	Tumor invasion of bladder and/or bowel mucosa
IVB*	Distant metastases, including intra-abdominal metastases and/or inguinal lymph nodes

* Either G1, G2 or G3.
** Endocervical glandular involvement only should be considered as Stage I and no longer as Stage II.
† Positive cytology has to be reported separately without changing the stage.

Table 7.2 FIGO staging of carcinoma of the endometrium. Reprinted from International Journal of Gynecology & Obstetrics 2009105: 103–104. Pecorelli S, Revised FIGO staging for carcinoma of the vulva, cervix, and endometrium, with permission from Elsevier.

sentinel nodes has been lower than other gynecologic malignancies, and pelvic lymph node dissection is not currently standard care.[8]

A possible entity that may be confused with endometrial adenocarcinoma, particularly on curettage specimens, is microglandular hyperplasia of the endocervix, which is less atypical and mitotic. Endometrioid histology can also occur in a primary endocervical carcinoma. Although the results may not be conclusive, an endometrial primary is more likely to be positive for vimentin and estrogen receptor, and negative for CEA, whereas the reverse is true for an endocervical primary;[19] however, CEA often is not helpful. HPV detection by in situ hybridization, or a marker of HPV such as p16, may confirm an endocervical primary, although it is not detectable in all cases.[9,20]

One of the most problematic areas is the distinction between atypical hyperplasia and endometrioid carcinoma on curettage specimens. Kurman and Norris identified their definition of stromal invasion as the feature most predictive of carcinoma at hysterectomy.[21] They defined stromal invasion as infiltration into a desmoplastic stroma, cribriform and confluent glands with no intervening stroma, an extensive papillary pattern, or replacement of the stroma by masses of squamous epithelium, the last three criteria having to occupy at least 2.1 mm (half of a low-power field 4.2 mm in diameter).[21] Silverberg[22] defined stromal invasion as stromal disappearance, desmoplasia or necrosis. The two features that have been found to be most reliable are degree of complexity of glandular architecture, and degree of atypia. Based on these two aspects, McKenny et al[23] proposed stratification of problematic endometrial proliferation into a three-tiered system based on risk of myoinvasion at hysterectomy: complex atypical hyperplasia with < 0.05% risk, complex atypical hyperplasia, cannot exclude well-differentiated adenocarcinoma (borderline), with a 5.5% risk, and well differentiated adenocarcinoma with a 20% risk.

Variants of endometrioid adenocarcinoma

Villoglandular

The villoglandular variant of endometrioid carcinoma (**Figure 7.6**) architecturally resembles a villous adenoma of the colon. For lesions

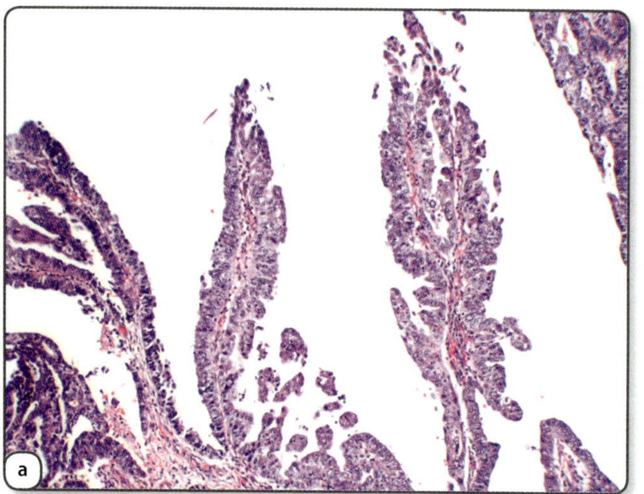

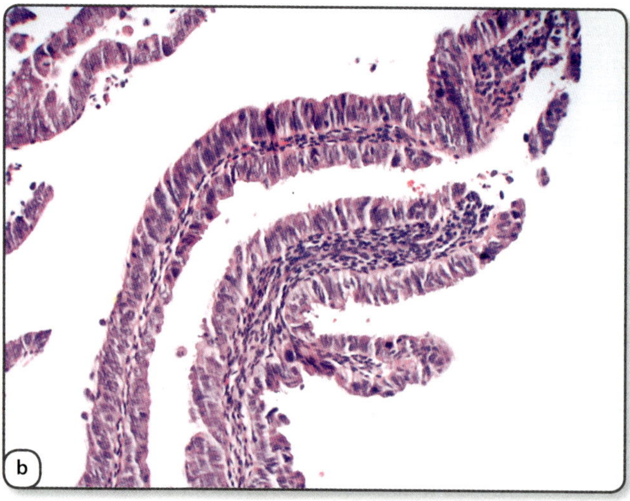

Figure 7.6 Villoglandular variant of endometrioid adenocarcinoma. The villous structures are more delicate and narrow than in serous carcinoma (a), and higher power shows the lack of degree of nuclear atypia expected in serous carcinoma (b).

confined to the endometrium the prognosis is the same as for usual endometrioid carcinoma, although it has been suggested that once myometrial invasion is present, villoglandular tumors are more aggressive.[24] The main differential is uterine serous carcinoma with a papillary architecture. The villous structures are more delicate and narrow in villoglandular carcinoma than in serous carcinoma, with thin fibrovascular cores, and they do not show the degree of nuclear atypia seen in serous carcinoma. The villoglandular change may only be focal or it may be diffuse. The cytology is similar to usual endometrioid carcinoma. The differentials include an uncommon lesion: a focal benign papillary change with bland cytology that was most often associated with endometrial polyps in the series of Lehman and Hart.[25]

Endometrioid carcinoma with squamous differentiation

Endometrioid adenocarcinoma with squamous differentiation (**Figure 7.7**) represents about 25% of endometrioid carcinomas.[9] The squamous foci may appear as morules, or as more solid areas, either keratinizing or not, or as individual keratinized cells. Sometimes there is spindling of the cells as well. The areas may blend imperceptibly with the glandular foci, making them appear more solid than they are and allowing the possibility of upgrading. Squamous differentiation used to be split into adenoacanthomas for lesions with well-differentiated histologically bland squamous foci, and adenosquamous carcinoma for lesions with histologically malignant squamous foci. However the differentiation tends to parallel the glandular differentiation, upon which the grade is based. The preferred term is adenocarcinoma with squamous differentiation. Some pathologists prefer to use the terminology of “adenoacanthoma” and “adenosquamous carcinoma” for curettage/biopsy specimens, to alert the clinician to the possibility that a more aggressive neoplasm (in the case of adenosquamous carcinoma) may be present prior to hysterectomy. In cases where the squamous differentiation is not clear-cut, the criteria for identification include keratinization demonstrable with standard staining techniques, intercellular bridges, or three of the following four criteria:[22]

- sheet-like growth without glands or palisading
- sharp cell margins
- eosinophilic/thick/glassy cytoplasm
- a decreased nuclear-to-cytoplasmic ratio compared with the rest of the tumor.

Secretory adenocarcinoma

Endometrioid adenocarcinoma may at times have focal secretory features, with subnuclear or supranuclear vacuoles. Diffuse secretory change is uncommon[9] (**Figure 7.8a** and **b**). In premenopausal women, secretory adenocarcinoma is most often seen in the presence of a corpus luteum, which is exerting a transient progestational effect on the carcinoma. In postmenopausal women, endogenous or exogenous progesterone effect may be present; however, this may not be identifiable. The change

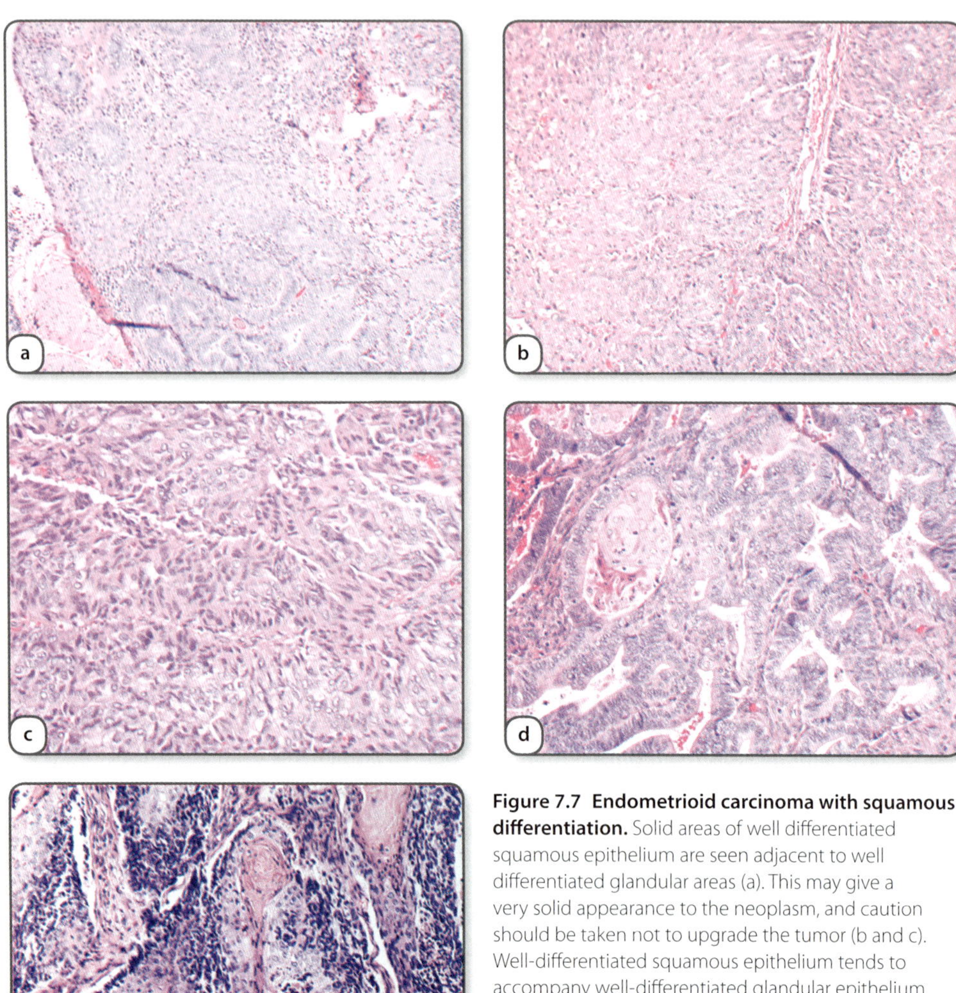

Figure 7.7 Endometrioid carcinoma with squamous differentiation. Solid areas of well differentiated squamous epithelium are seen adjacent to well differentiated glandular areas (a). This may give a very solid appearance to the neoplasm, and caution should be taken not to upgrade the tumor (b and c). Well-differentiated squamous epithelium tends to accompany well-differentiated glandular epithelium (d), and high-grade squamous epithelium tends to accompany more poorly differentiated tumors (e).

may be transient and seen at curettage but not persisting to the time of hysterectomy. Prognosis is the same as for usual endometrioid carcinoma. The main differential is clear cell adenocarcinoma, which is more likely to be either solid or papillary, to have clearing of the cytoplasm, to lack subnuclear or supranuclear vacuoles, and to have a greater degree of nuclear atypia than secretory carcinoma.[9]

Ciliated adenocarcinoma

This rare variant is thought to have a similar prognosis to usual endometrioid adenocarcinoma, and has foci composed almost entirely or entirely of ciliated cells.[9]

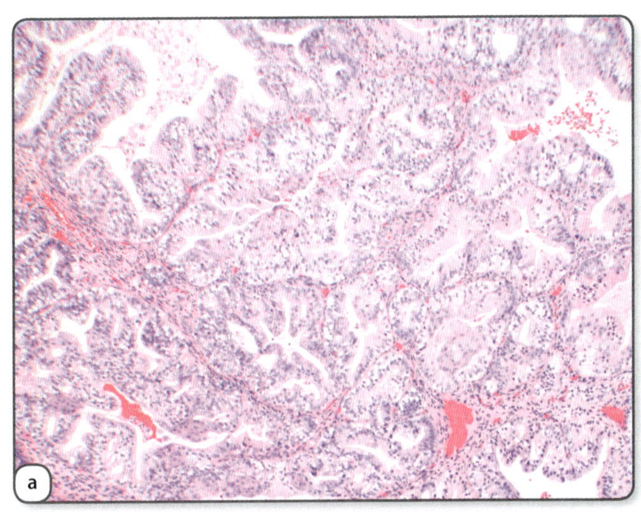

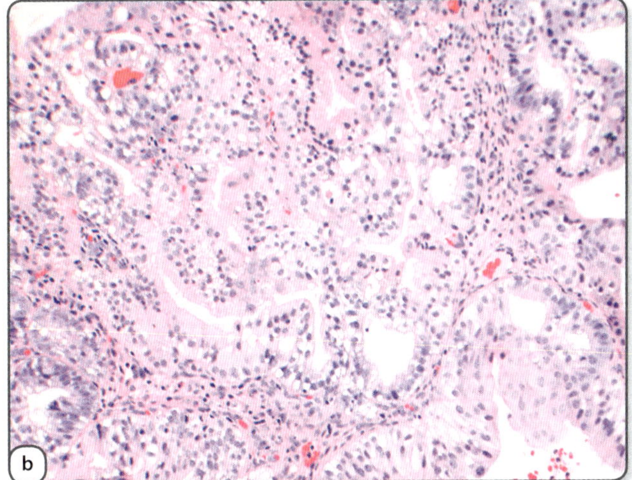

Figure 7.8 Secretory carcinoma. The adenocarcinoma has subnuclear vacuoles, mimicking a day-17 secretory endometrium. Note focal squamous metaplasia as well.

Nonendometrioid adenocarcinoma

Uterine serous carcinoma

Uterine serous carcinomas represent 5–10% of endometrial carcinomas.[5] Although occasionally associated with tamoxifen or radiation, most have no such associations, and are not related to the hyperestrogenic pathway.[5] The tumors are often advanced at surgical staging, with a propensity to spread in a manner similar to ovarian serous carcinomas, involving peritoneal surfaces, omentum, and pelvic and para-aortic lymph nodes.

The tumors may be papillary in configuration with fibrovascular cores, hence the older term "uterine papillary serous carcinoma". However, the tumor may form glandular or solid patterns as well (**Figure 7.9**). The cytology is the striking feature, with marked atypia,

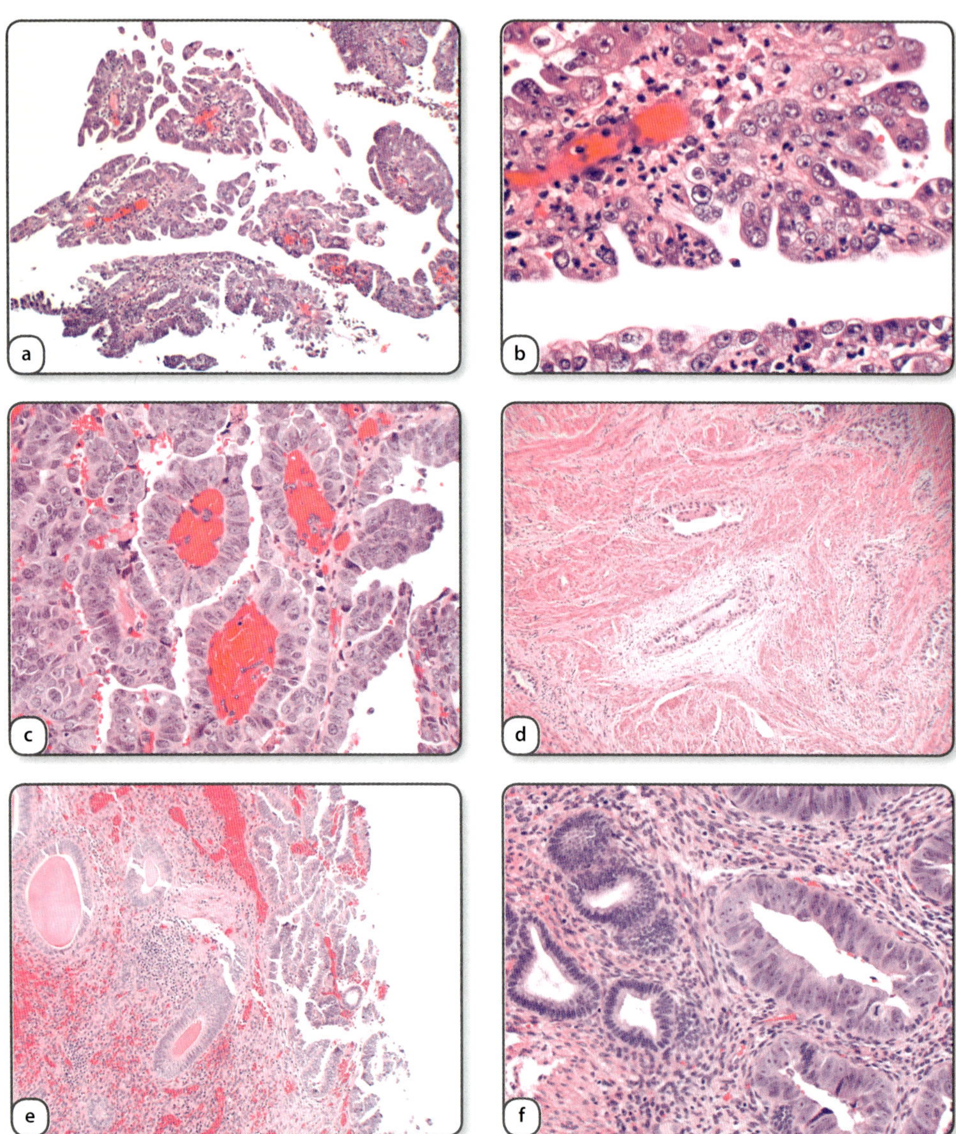

Figure 7.9 Uterine serous carcinoma. When papillary in configuration (a), the papillae are thicker and blunter than the villoglandular variant of endometrioid. Fibrovascular cores are lined by a markedly atypical epithelium showing nuclear pleomorphism with prominent nucleoli (b and c). Uterine serous often invades by individual glands rather than a pushing tumor front (d), and early lymphvascular invasion is common. It may be confined to the surface epithelium (e), and still show widespread metastatic disease. Serous nuclei on the right are larger than normal nuclei on the left (f), and show prominent nucleoli. The tumor may show a more solid pattern (g). Superimposed progestin effect on an unexpected serous carcinoma (h) and (i) shows preservation of the glandular atypia within a decidualized stroma. Serous tumors may also assume an endometrioid glandular architecture, but the nuclear features are serous. In indeterminate cases (j), immunohistochemistry staining for p53 and p16 may help with the distinction.

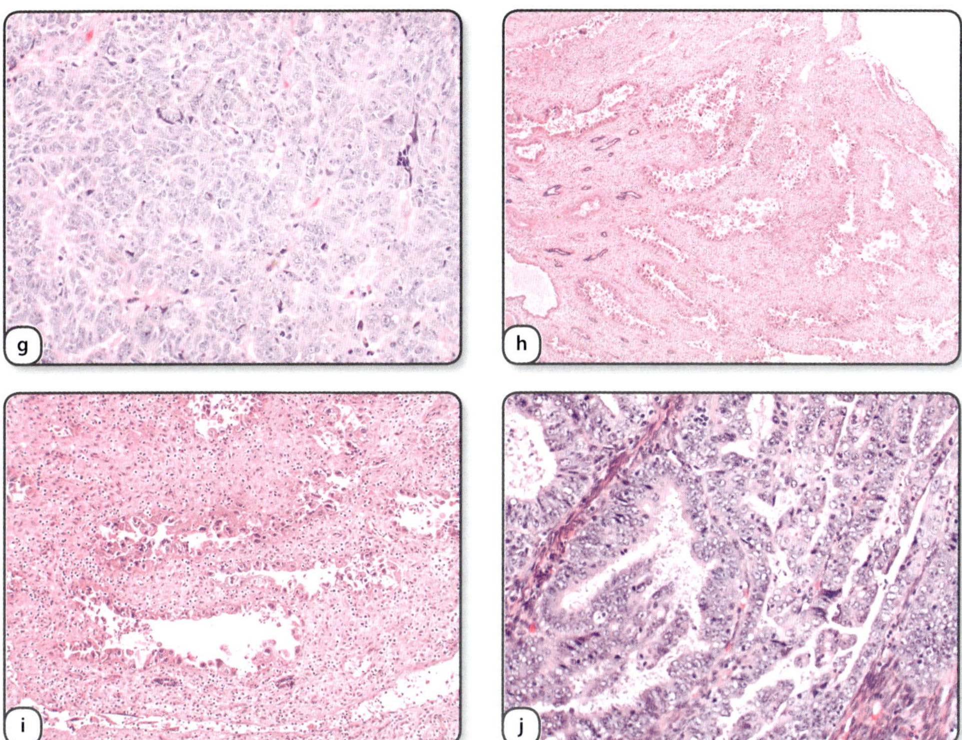

Figure 7.9 Uterine serous carcinoma. ***Continued.***

pleomorphism, mitotic activity, and large nucleoli. Early carcinomas may arise in an endometrial polyp and even in such a case, or without myometrial invasion, there is often extensive lymphvascular involvement in the uterus. Surface involvement by EIC may be seen adjacent in many cases and, as mentioned previously, EIC in isolation can metastasize (see Chapter 6). Serous carcinomas are not graded,[10] and are all considered grade 3.

The differential diagnosis of serous carcinoma includes papillary syncytial change, radiation atypia, villoglandular endometrioid carcinoma, clear cell carcinoma with a papillary pattern, and metastatic serous carcinoma from the ovaries, fallopian tubes or peritoneum.

Differentiating serous from endometrioid carcinoma

A carcinoma with a glandular architecture and marked nuclear atypia raises the differential of an endometrioid adenocarcinoma requiring upgrading based on nuclei, or a serous carcinoma with a glandular architecture. This is a difficult area, with no single immunohistochemical stain that will consistently distinguish between the two, and hence a panel is more likely to be helpful.[10] p53 favors, but is not diagnostic of, serous carcinoma as some serous carcinomas are negative and some high-grade endometrioid carcinomas are positive. Estrogen and progesterone receptor positivity (ER/PR) favor endometrioid carcinoma. Serous carcinomas have higher Ki-67 indices than low-grade endometrioid carcinomas; however, high-grade endometrioid carcinomas will show intermediate values. Phosphatase and tensin homologue (PTEN) is more often lost in endometrioid carcinomas. Overall, serous carcinomas show much stronger diffuse staining with p16.[10] Clarke et al recommend a panel of p53, ER, PTEN, and p16 to distinguish endometrioid from serous carcinoma.[10] Overlap is a potential issue, with high-grade endometrioid carcinomas exhibiting overlapping immunoprofiles as well as morphology with serous carcinomas.[25]

Clear cell adenocarcinoma

Clear cell adenocarcinoma of the endometrium is uncommon, representing 1–6% of endometrial cancers.[26] Although often thought of as a more aggressive carcinoma, the literature is controversial.[27] Data suggest overall 5-year survival is lower than for endometrioid carcinoma.[28]

Histologically, the lesions are similar in appearance to clear cell tumors of other organs such as kidney. There may be solid or glandular areas composed of clear cells, or the tumor may be tubulopapillary with hobnailed cells, which may also have clear cytoplasm (**Figure 7.10**). Clear cell carcinomas are not graded,[10] and are all considered grade 3 by definition.

Similar to serous carcinomas, clear cell carcinomas are negative for ER/PR, and have a high Ki-67 index, but they are much less p53 positive than serous carcinomas.[29]

Much less is known about the molecular basis of clear cell carcinoma than serous carcinoma, probably related to the relative rarity of the former. Fadare et al[26] described a putative precursor lesion, which was identified adjacent to clear cell carcinomas in the benign endometrium and had an intermediate immunoprofile between normal and clear cell when evaluated with ER/PR, p53, and Ki-67. An et al suggested that there may be more than one pathway for clear cell carcinomas, as mixed carcinomas showed similar p53 and PTEN mutations and microsatellite instability in both clear cell and non-clear cell components of the lesion, whereas p53 and PTEN mutations were rare in pure clear cell carcinoma.[27]

The differential diagnosis includes metastatic clear cell carcinoma from an extrauterine site, Arias-Stella reaction, and hobnail metaplasia for the hobnail patterns, and secretory carcinoma and squamous cell carcinoma with cytoplasmic clearing for the more solid clear cell tumors.

Squamous cell carcinoma

Pure squamous cell carcinoma of the endometrium is exceptionally rare (**Figure 7.11**). Squamous differentiation within a glandular

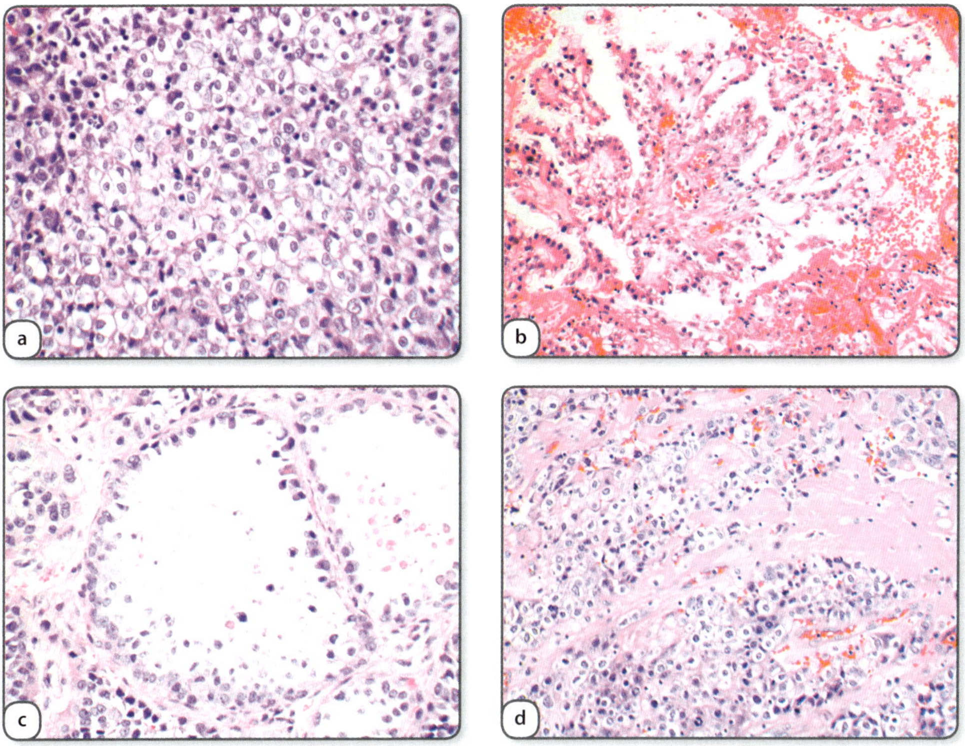

Figure 7.10 Clear cell adenocarcinoma. The lesion may be composed of clear cells in a solid (a), glandular, or papillary (b) configuration, or may be tubulopapillary (c). Abundant eosinophilic fibrinoid material is often seen, and is a possible clue to the tumor type (d).

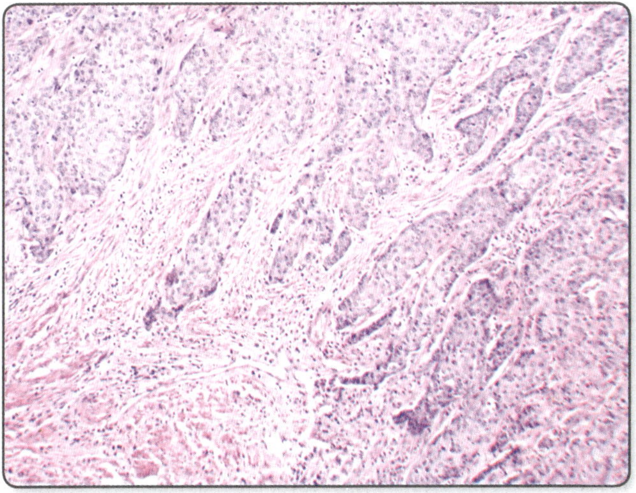

Figure 7.11 Squamous cell carcinoma of the endometrium.

lesion, or spread from a primary cervical neoplasm should always be considered first. Associations with pure squamous cell carcinoma of the endometrium include longstanding pyometra, cervical stenosis, uterine prolapse, squamous metaplasia, and a history of radiation.[9] The criteria established by Fluhmann in 1928[30] are still applicable and include that there is no coexisting endometrial adenocarcinoma, no connection to the cervical squamous epithelium, and no coexisting primary squamous cell carcinoma of the cervix. In addition, the WHO has added that there must be keratinization or intracellular bridges seen in the tumor.[31] The differential diagnosis of squamous cell carcinoma of the endometrium includes benign squamous metaplasia, endometrioid adenocarcinoma with extensive squamous differentiation, decidua, placental site nodule/plaque, placental site trophoblastic tumor, epithelioid trophoblastic tumor and spread from a cervical squamous cell carcinoma.

Mucinous adenocarcinoma

Endometrial carcinomas of endometrioid type may have mucinous foci. Different studies vary in the amount of mucinous epithelium needed to be able to call a carcinoma a mucinous adenocarcinoma, with the WHO requiring 90%.[9] The architecture of mucinous adenocarcinoma is similar to that of endometrioid carcinomas. The cytological features are often show minimal or no atypia (**Figure 7.12**), making the distinction from a benign process more difficult.

The differential diagnosis includes mucinous metaplasia of the endometrium. This can be a difficult distinction, particularly on curettage, given the lack of atypia seen in many mucinous adenocarcinomas. Admixture with normal benign endometrium should be sought to make the distinction. Other lesions in the differential include normal endocervical tissue in curettings, microglandular hyperplasia, mucinous endocervical adenocarcinoma, and metastatic mucinous carcinoma.

Mixed carcinoma

When an endometrioid carcinoma has a significant component of a second cell type (defined as over 10%), it is categorized as a mixed carcinoma.[9]

Transitional cell carcinoma (TCC)

Pure transitional cell carcinomas of the endometrium are exceptionally rare, with experience predominantly limited to case reports.[32] The WHO requires at least 90% of the tumor to be transitional for a designation of TCC, with lesser degrees considered to be mixed carcinomas with transitional differentiation.[1] Histologically, the tumor resembles TCC elsewhere, and the differential includes metastasis of TCC from another site, squamous cell carcinoma, particularly if papillary, as well as undifferentiated carcinoma. Cases are too few for specific treatment or prognostic recommendations.[32]

Small cell carcinoma

Small cell carcinoma with neuroendocrine differentiation is rare in the endometrium, and may be either a pure pattern or mixed with other tumor types. Histologically it resembles small cell carcinoma of the lung. Although the lesion appears to be more aggressive than

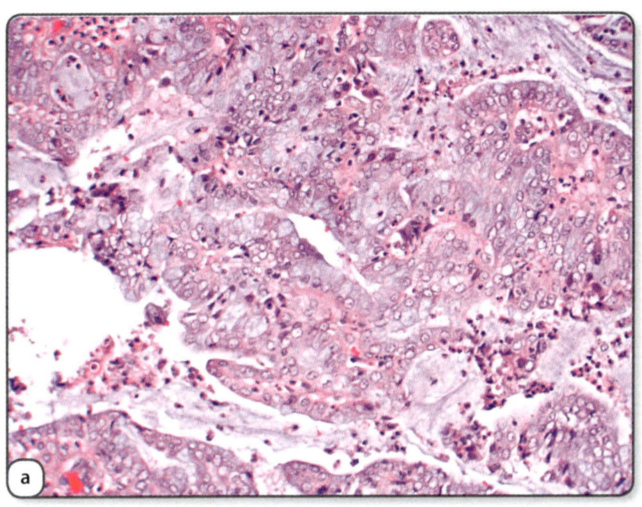

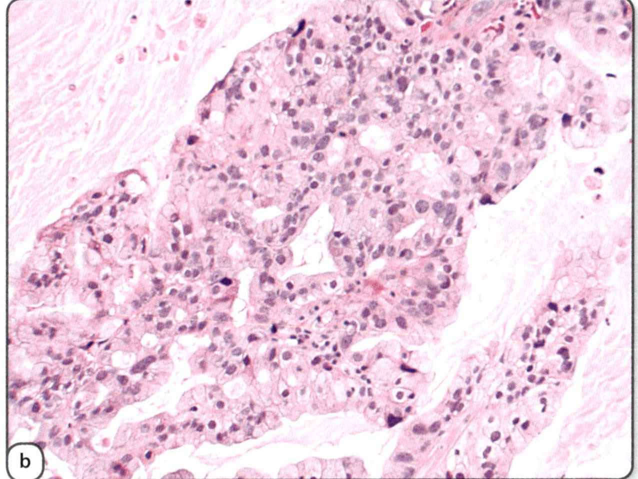

Figure 7.12 Mucinous adenocarcinoma may be focal (a) or diffuse (b).

endometrioid adenocarcinoma, it has a 5-year survival of about 60% for stage I disease.[1] It may be associated with paraneoplastic syndromes such as Cushing syndrome, hypoglycemia, inappropriate secretion of anti-diuretic hormone, visual disturbances and membranous glomerulonephritis.[33]

Undifferentiated carcinoma

Undifferentiated carcinoma of the endometrium (**Figure 7.13**) is distinguished from FIGO grade 3 endometrioid adenocarcinoma by total lack of either glandular or squamous differentiation.[34] The prognosis is worse for undifferentiated carcinoma than endometrioid.[34] The solid areas lack any hint of gland formation, unlike grade 3 endometrioid (which has areas of glands), which even in the solid area has trabeculae or cords of cells resembling the glandular cells. Keratin and epithelial membrane antigen (EMA) are less likely to be positive in undifferentiated

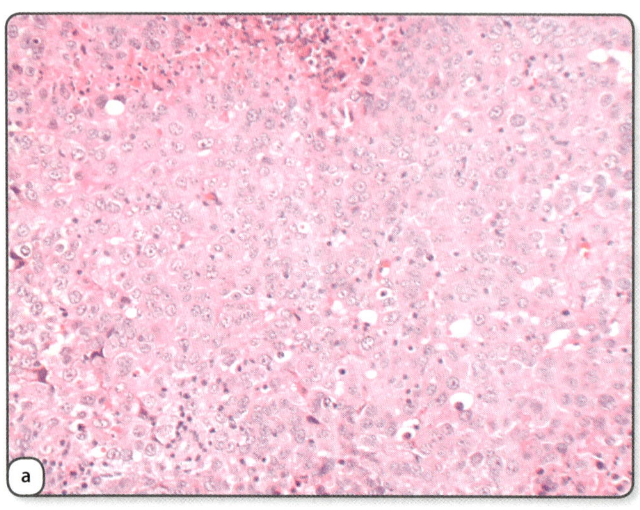

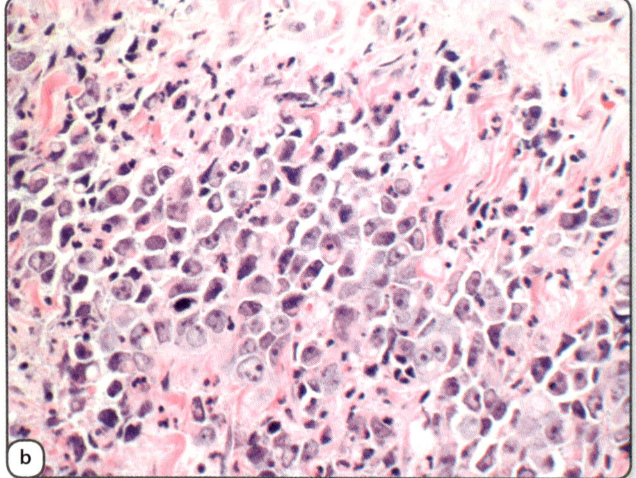

Figure 7.13 Undifferentiated carcinoma shows no features of any specific tumor type, as seen in this endometrial tumor (a), and peritoneal implant (b).

carcinomas.[34] It has been suggested that undifferentiated or dedifferentiated endometrial carcinomas (with undifferentiated foci adjacent to glandular foci) is a risk factor for Lynch syndrome.[35]

Mixed epithelial and mesenchymal malignancies

Carcinosarcoma (malignant mixed müllerian or mesodermal tumor)

After recognition of the overlap between the immunoprofiles of the carcinomatous and sarcomatous portions of the lesion, the current thinking is that carcinosarcomas represent metaplastic carcinomas, with biphasic histology (**Figure 7.14**). The patients are usually postmenopausal and often about 10 years older than the usual patient

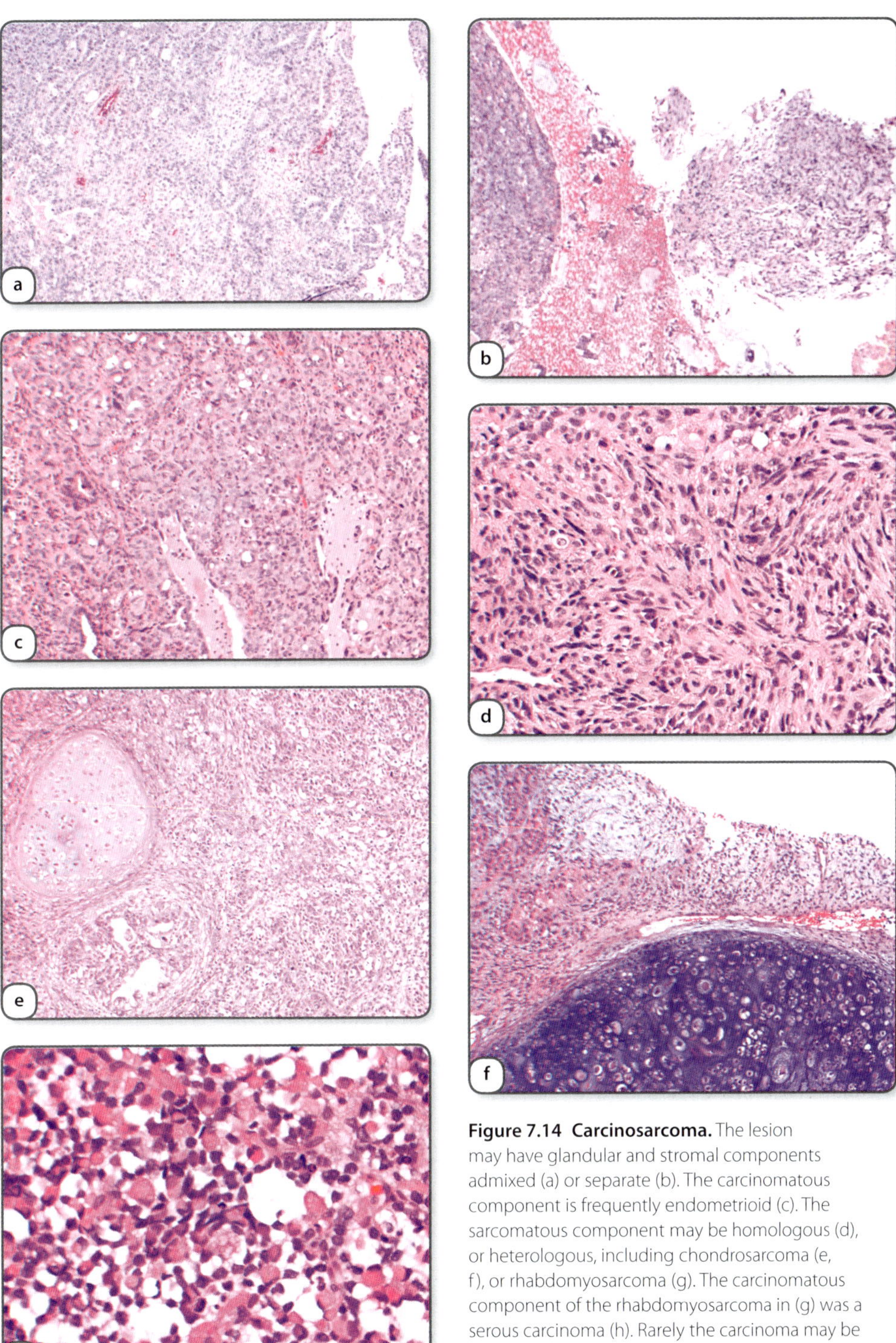

Figure 7.14 Carcinosarcoma. The lesion may have glandular and stromal components admixed (a) or separate (b). The carcinomatous component is frequently endometrioid (c). The sarcomatous component may be homologous (d), or heterologous, including chondrosarcoma (e, f), or rhabdomyosarcoma (g). The carcinomatous component of the rhabdomyosarcoma in (g) was a serous carcinoma (h). Rarely the carcinoma may be squamous (i).

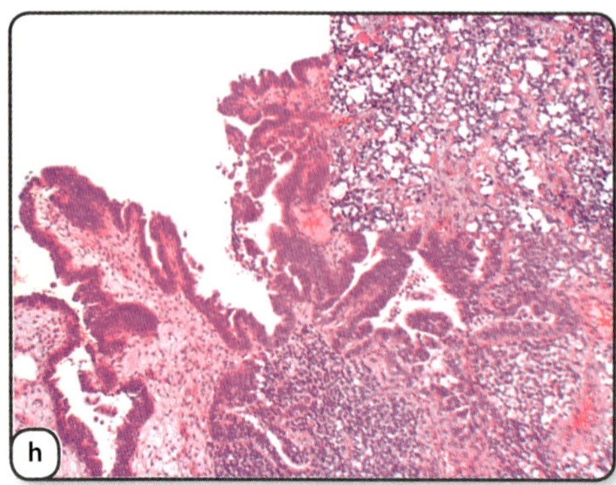

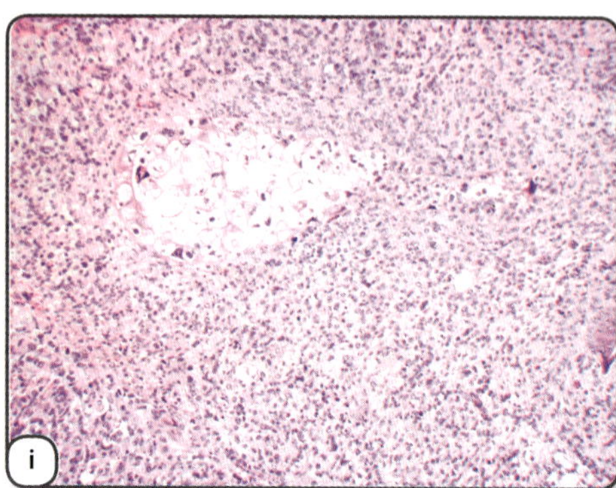

Figure 7.14 Carcinosarcoma. *Continued.*

with endometrial carcinoma. The tumors are often large and polypoid. Histologically, the carcinoma is most often endometrioid, but it may also be any other histology seen in the endometrium, including serous, and even squamous. The mesenchymal portion may be homologous (i.e. native to the uterus, such as leiomyosarcoma, stromal sarcoma, or undifferentiated sarcoma) or heterologous (such as chondrosarcoma or rhabdomyosarcoma), but this does not alter prognosis for this aggressive neoplasm.[36] Carcinosarcomas are staged with the same system as endometrial adenocarcinomas.

Müllerian adenosarcoma

Müllerian adenosarcomas are uncommon neoplasms, most often seen in the postmenopausal age group, although occurring in all age groups. Grossly, these are polypoid malignancies. Histologically, adenosarcomas are composed of benign glands within a malignant stroma (**Figure 7.15**). The stroma may be seen condensing around the glands forming a cambium layer,[37] or the tumor may assume a leaf-like pattern, with the benign epithelium lining "phyllodes-like" sarcomatous outgrowths. Typically the sarcomatous portion is low grade, and of endometrial stromal/fibroblastic type,[37] but it may be high grade, with sarcomatous overgrowth. If it is low grade, the immunoprofile is similar to stromal sarcomas, with positivity for ER, PR, CD10 and Wilms tumor protein (WT1), and low Ki-67 index.[37] Sex cord differentiation and/or heterologous elements may be seen. Adenosarcomas are staged with stromal sarcomas (**Table 7.3**).[38] They are usually low-grade malignancies, however prognosis worsens with sarcomatous overgrowth or deep myometrial invasion.[37]

Sarcomas of the uterus

Endometrial stromal tumors

Endometrial stromal neoplasms are composed of cells resembling the stroma of proliferative endometrium.[39] They are divided into

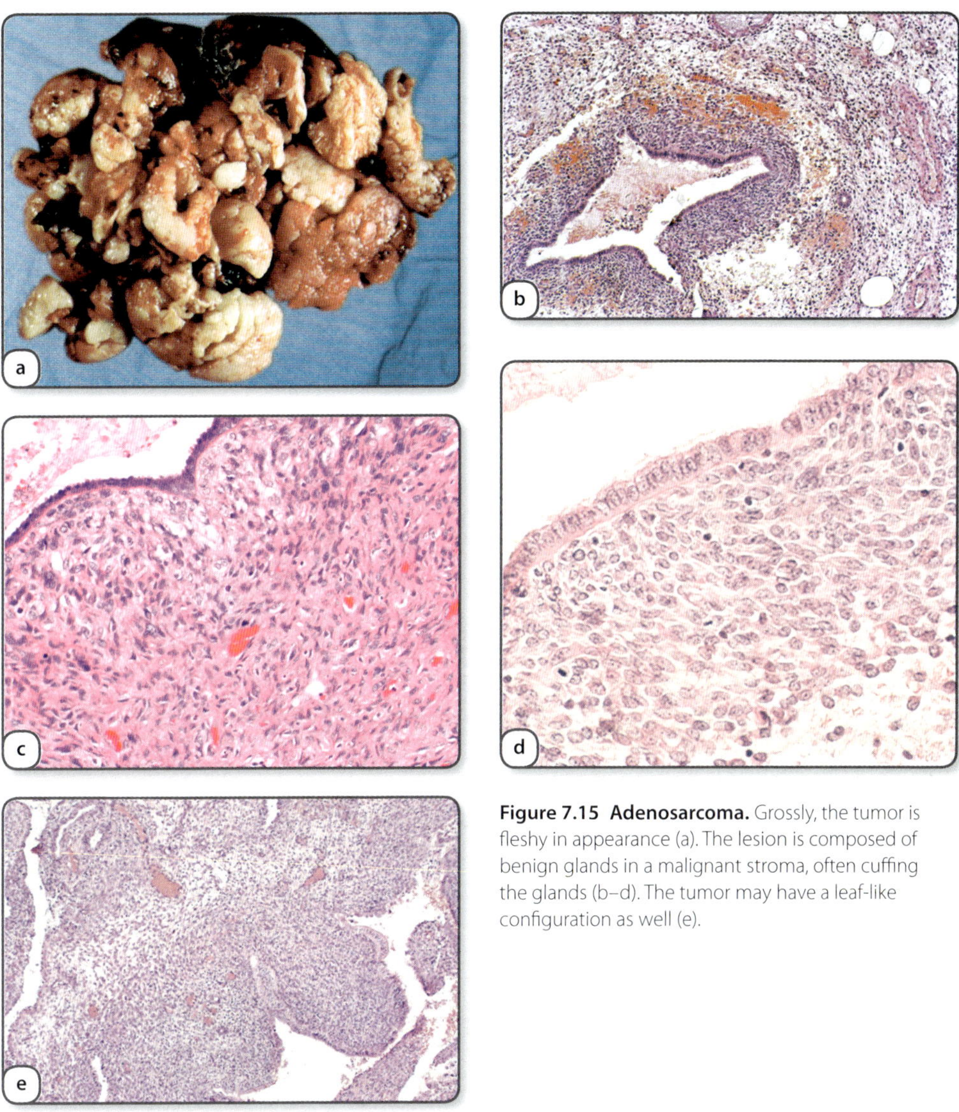

Figure 7.15 Adenosarcoma. Grossly, the tumor is fleshy in appearance (a). The lesion is composed of benign glands in a malignant stroma, often cuffing the glands (b–d). The tumor may have a leaf-like configuration as well (e).

benign endometrial stromal nodules, low-grade endometrial stromal sarcomas, and undifferentiated endometrial sarcomas.

Endometrial stromal sarcoma (low-grade endometrial stromal sarcoma, ESS)

Endometrial stromal sarcomas are uncommon but not rare, and they are seen most often in middle-aged women. There may be an association with a hyperestrogenic state. Grossly, the lesions often infiltrate the myometrium in worm-like tumor cords projecting from the cut surface of the myometrium. Histologically, the tumor resembles proliferative endometrial stroma, with prominent blood

FIGO staging for uterine sarcomas (2009)	
Stage	**Definition**
Leiomyosarcomas and endometrial stromal sarcomas*	
I	Tumor limited to uterus
IA	≤ to 5 cm
IB	> 5 cm
II	Tumor extends beyond the uterus, within the pelvis
IIA	Adnexal involvement
IIB	Involvement of other pelvic tissues
III	Tumor invades abdominal tissues (not just protruding into the abdomen)
IIIA	One site
IIIB	More than one site
IIIC	Metastasis to pelvic and/or para-aortic lymph nodes
IV	
IVA	Tumor invades bladder and/or rectum
IVB	Distant metastasis
Adenosarcomas	
I	Tumor limited to uterus
IA	Tumor limited to endometrium/endocervix with no myometrial invasion
IB	≤ half myometrial invasion
IC	More than half myometrial invasion
II	Tumor extends beyond the uterus, within the pelvis
IIA	Adnexal involvement
IIB	Tumor extends to extrauterine pelvic tissue
III	Tumor invades abdominal tissues (not just protruding into the abdomen)
IIIA	One site
IIIB	More than one site
IIIC	Metastasis to pelvic and/or para-aortic lymph nodes
IV	
IVA	Tumor invades bladder and/or rectum
IVB	Distant metastasis
Carcinosarcomas	
Should be staged as carcinomas of the endometrium	

* Note: Simultaneous endometrial stromal sarcomas of the uterine corpus and ovary/ pelvis in association with ovarian/ pelvic endometriosis should be classified as independent primary tumors.

Table 7.3 FIGO staging of endometrial stromal sarcomas and adenosarcomas. Reprinted from Gynecologic Oncology, 116, 2010 D'Angelo E, Prat J. Uterine Sarcomas: a review. p131–139, with permission from Elsevier.

vessels (**Figure 7.16**). Atypia is minimal, necrosis not usual, and mitotic activity is usually less than 5 mitoses per 10 high-power fields. The tumors, as well as stromal nodules (see p. 118) stain for vimentin, smooth muscle actin, and usually CD 10. As this immunoprofile may be the same in a smooth muscle neoplasm, often in the differential, a negative h-caldesmon in a stromal lesion may be helpful.[39] These low-grade malignancies are characterized by late recurrences, so

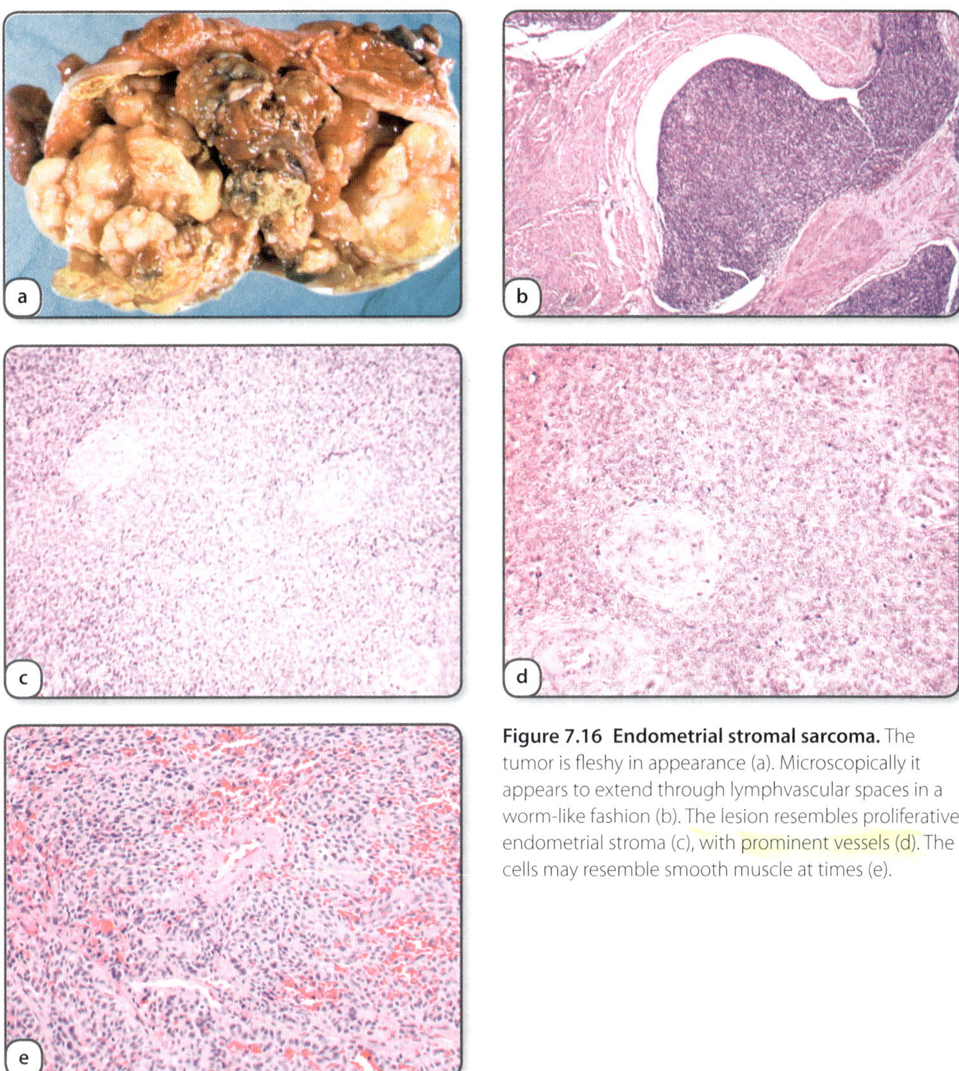

Figure 7.16 Endometrial stromal sarcoma. The tumor is fleshy in appearance (a). Microscopically it appears to extend through lymphvascular spaces in a worm-like fashion (b). The lesion resembles proliferative endometrial stroma (c), with prominent vessels (d). The cells may resemble smooth muscle at times (e).

prolonged follow-up is necessary. Stromal sarcomas are staged with adenosarcomas (**Table 7.3**).[38]

Glandular elements may occasionally be seen in ESS, and hence the differential includes an adenosarcoma. Adenosarcomas tend to have greater numbers of larger glands, with cuffing of the mesenchymal portion of the lesion around those glands. If the sarcoma of adenosarcoma resembles ESS, or if the glands of an ESS are more numerous, it may be very difficult to distinguish the two lesions. The biologic behavior of both is similar, i.e. indolent, and hence it becomes less critical to make the distinction between the two in difficult cases.[40] This diagnostic difficulty is rare.[41] Frequently ESS has a t(11;17) translocation.[41]

Stromal nodule

Stromal nodules are benign lesions histologically similar to low-grade stromal sarcomas, but they are distinguished by their lack of infiltration (**Figure 7.17**). They may be endometrial or myometrial in location. Occasional projections may be seen into adjacent myometrium but should not exceed 3.[39] Hysterectomy is curative. On curettage specimens, it is essentially impossible to distinguish stromal nodule from ESS, and hence the diagnosis is almost always made at hysterectomy.

Undifferentiated endometrial sarcoma

Undifferentiated sarcomas of the endometrium are markedly pleomorphic neoplasms with brisk mitotic activity and possible necrosis[39] (**Figure 7.18**). They resemble the sarcomatous portion of a carcinosarcoma, and adequate sampling to rule out that more common neoplasm by finding a carcinomatous region should be undertaken. They are infiltrative rather than forming the worm-like plugs of ESS. Undifferentiated sarcomas are staged with ESS and adenosarcomas (**Table 3.3**).[38]

Metastatic carcinoma

The most common tumors that metastasize to the endometrium are those from other genital organs, the fallopian tubes, ovaries, and cervix; however, a variety of other carcinomas can spread to the endometrium as well, particularly the colon, stomach, and breast[9] (**Figure 7.19**). In the case of a pure mucinous adenocarcinoma in the endometrium, a cervical primary must be considered. Preservation of benign endometrial glands between tumor, extensive lymphvascular involvement, greater myometrial than endometrial involvement, and a multinodular or infiltrative pattern are features than should raise consideration of metastatic disease.[9]

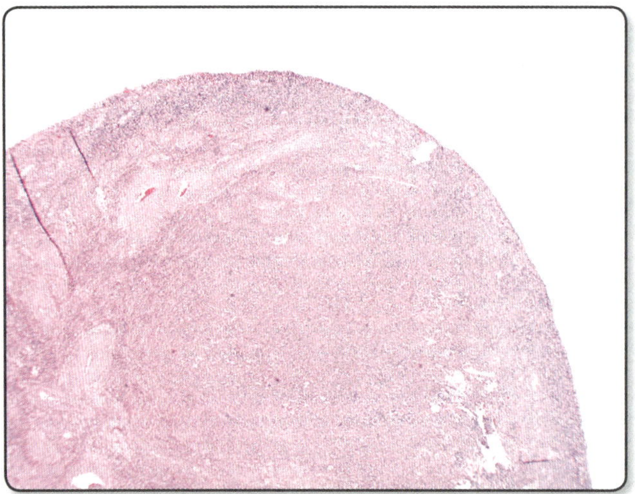

Figure 7.17 Stromal nodule. Lack of invasion of this polypoid lesion is what distinguishes this lesion from endometrial stromal sarcoma.

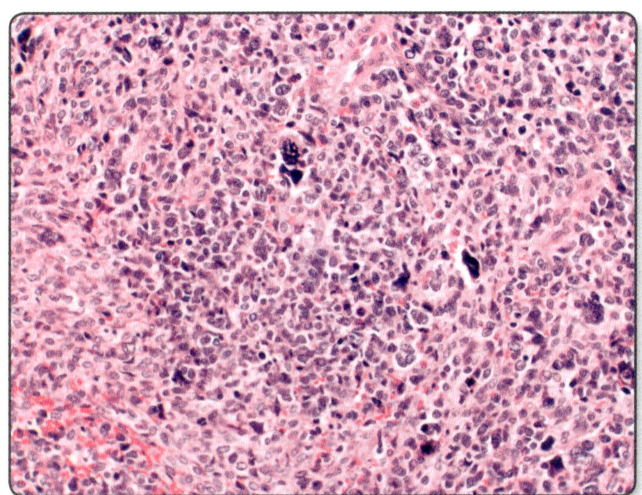

Figure 7.18 Undifferentiated sarcoma showing marked pleomorphism.

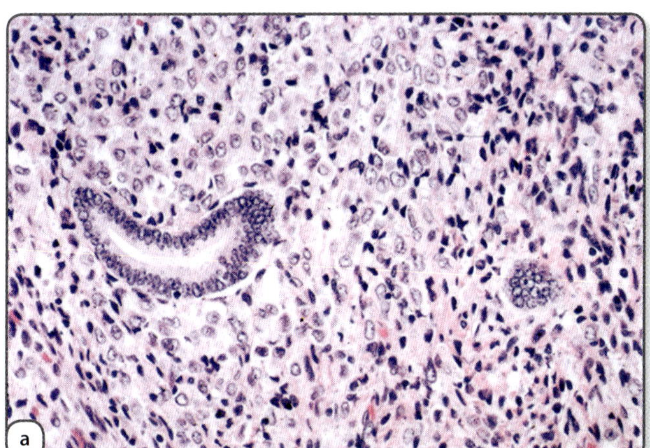

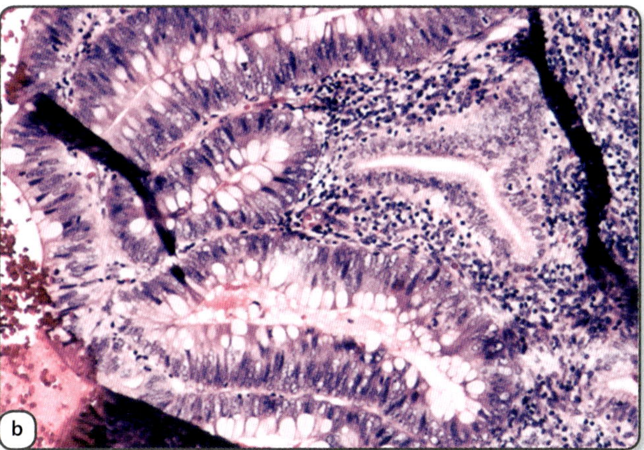

Figure 7.19 Metastatic carcinoma. Metastatic breast carcinoma sparing benign glands (a). Metastatic colon cancer (b) on a curettage, admixed with benign endometrial tissue.

Problems with artifacts

Individual artifacts are discussed in the next chapter. However, it is notable that uterine manipulation may increase artifacts and complicate cancer diagnoses. Based on personal experience, this includes rough handling of the uterine specimen, which may displace tumor. A recent study[42] attributed increased rates of disruption of the endometrial lining, nuclear crush artifact, vascular pseudoinvasion, endomyometrial cleft artifact with or without epithelial displacement, inflammatory debris within vessels, serosal carryover, intratubal contaminants and increased rates of positive peritoneal washings to laparoscopically assisted hysterectomies in which uterine manipulators were utilized, hampering pathologic interpretation and increasing adjuvant study usage.

References

1. Tavassoli RA, Devilee P, eds. Tumors of the Breast and Female Genital Tract Organs. World Health Organization Classification of Tumors. Lyon, Washington DC, IARC Press, 2003.
2. Deligdisch L, Holinka CF. Endometrial carcinoma: two diseases? Cancer Detect Prev 1987;10:237–46.
3. Westhoff C, Heller D, Drosinos S, Tancer L. Risk factors for hyperplasia-associated versus atrophy-associated endometrial carcinoma. Am J Obstet Gynecol 2000 ;182:506–08.
4. Sherman ME, Devesa SS. Analysis of racial differences in incidence, survival, and mortality for malignant tumors of the uterine corpus. Cancer 2003;98:176–86.
5. Clement PB, Young RH. Non-endometrioid carcinomas of the uterine corpus: a review of their pathology with emphasis on recent advances and problematic aspects. Adv Anat Pathol 2004;11:117–42.
6. Arafa M, Somja J, Dehan P, Kridelka F, Goffin F, et al. Current concepts in the pathology and epigenetics of endometrial carcinoma. Pathol 2010;42:613–17.
7. Hunn J, Dodson MK, Webb J, Soisson AP. Endometrial cancer – current state of the art therapies and unmet clinical needs: the role of surgery and preoperative radiographic assessment. Adv Drug Deliv Rev 2009;61:890–95.
8. Oonk MH, van de Nieuwenhof HP, de Hullu JA, van der Zee AG. The role of sentinel node biopsy in gynecological cancer: a review. Curr Op Oncol 2009;21:425–32.
9. Clement PB, Young RH. Endometrioid carcinoma of the uterine corpus: a review of its pathology with emphasis on recent advances and problematic aspects. Adv Anat Pathol 2002;9:145–84.
10. Clarke BA, Gilks CB. Endometrial carcinoma: controversies in histopathological assessment of grade and tumor cell type. J Clin Pathol 2010;63:410–15.
11. Heller D, Drosinos S, Westhoff C. Accuracy of tumor grade assigned at initial endometrial sampling. Int J Gynecol Obstet, 1994; 47:301–02.
12. Alkushi A, Abdul-Rahman ZH, Lim P, Schulzer M, Coldman A, et al. Description of a novel system for grading of endometrial carcinoma and comparison with existing grading systems. Am J Surg Pathol 2005;29:295–304.
13. Ali A, Black D, Soslow RA. Difficulties in assessing the depth of myometrial invasion in endometrial carcinoma. Int J Gynecol Pathol 2007;26:115–23.
14. Creaseman W. Revised FIGO staging for carcinoma of the endometrium. Int J Gynecol Obstet 2009;105:109.
15. FIGO Committee on Gynecologic Oncology. Revised FIGO staging for carcinoma of the vulva, cervix, and endometrium. Int J Gynecol Obstet 2009;105:103–04.
16. Jacques SM, Lawrence WD. Endometrial adenocarcinoma with variable-level myometrial involvement limited to adenomyosis: a clinicopathologic study of 23 cases. Gynecol Oncol 1990;37:401–07.
17. Nascimento AF, Hirsch MS, Cviko A, Quade BJ, Nucci MR. The role of CD10 staining in distinguishing invasive endometrial adenocarcinoma from adenocarcinoma involving adenomyosis. Mod Pathol 2003;16:22–27.

18. Kir G, Kir M, Cetiner H, Karateke A, Grbuz A. Diagnostic problems on frozen section examination of myometrial invasion in patients with endometrial carcinoma with special emphasis on the pitfalls of deep adenoyosis with carcinomatous involvement. Eur J Gynaecol Oncol 2004;25:211–14.
19. Zaino RJ. The fruits of our labors: distinguishing endometrial from endocervical adenocarcinoma. Int J Gynecol Pathol 2002;21:1–3.
20. Kong CS, Beck AH, Longacre TA. A panel of 3 markers including p16, ProExC, or HPV ISH is optimal for distinguishing between primary endometrial and endocervical adenocarcinomas. Am J Surg Pathol. 2010;34:915–26.
21. Kurman RJ, Norris HJ. Evaluation of criteria for distinguishing atypical endometrial hyperplasia from well-differentiated carcinoma. Cancer 1982;49:2547–59.
22. Silverberg SG. Problems in the differential diagnosis of endometrial hyperplasia and carcinoma. Mod Pathol 2000;13:309–27.
23. McKenney JK, Longacre TA. Low grade endometrial adenocarcinoma. A diagnostic algorithm for distinguishing atypical endometrial hyperplasia and other benign (and malignant) mimics. Adv Anat Pathol 2009;16:1–22.
24. Ambros RA, Ballouk F, Malfetano JH et al. Significance of papillary (villoglandular) differentiation in endometrioid carcinoma of the uterus. Am J Surg Pathol 1994;18:569–75.
25. Zannoni GF, Vellone VG, Arena V, Prisco MG, Scambia G, et al. Does high-grade endometrioid carcinoma (grade 3 FIGO) belong to type I or type II cancer? A clinical-pathological and immunohistochemical study. Virchows Archiv 2010;457:27–34.
26. Fadare O, Liang SX, Ulukus EC, Chambers SK, Zheng W. Precursors of endometrial clear cell carcinoma. Am J Surg Pathol 2006;30:1519–30.
27. An HJ, Logani S, Isacson C, Ellenson LH. Molecular characterization of uterine clear cell carcinoma. Mod Pathol 2004;17:530–37.
28. Gadducci A, Cosio S, Spirito N, Cionini L. Clear cell carcinoma of the endometrium: a biological and clinical enigma. Anticancer Res 2010; 30:1327–34.
29. Lax SF, Pizer ES, Ronnett BM, Kurman RJ. Clear cell carcinoma of the endometrium is characterized by a distinctive profile of p53, Ki-67, estrogen and progesterone receptor expression. Hum Pathol 1998;29:551–58.
30. Fluhmann CF Squamous epithelium in the endometrium in benign and malignant conditions. Surg Gynecol Obstet 1928;46:309–16.
31. Thomakos N, Galaal K, Godfrey KA, Hemming D, Naik R, et al. Primary endometrial squamous cell carcinoma. Arch Gynecol Obstet 2008; 278:177–80.
32. Marino-Enriquez A, Gonzalez-Rocha T, Burgos E, Stolnicu S, Mendiola M, et al. Transitional cell carcinoma of the endometrium and endometrial carcinoma with transitional cell differentiation: a clinicopathologic study of 5 cases and review of the literature. Hum Pathol 2008; 39:1606–13.
33. Albores-Saavedra J, Martinez-Benitez B, Luevano E. Small cell carcinomas and large cell neuroendocrine carcinomas of the endometrium and cervix: polypoid tumors and those arising in polyps may have a favorable prognosis. Int J Gynecol Pathol 2008; 27:333–39.
34. Altrabulsi B, Malpica A, Deavers MT, Bodurka, DC, Broaddus R, Silva EG. Undifferentiated carcinoma of the endometrium. Am J Surg Pathol 2005;25:52–58.
35. Garg K, Leitao MM Jr, Kauff ND, Hansen J, Kosarin K, Shia J, Soslow RA. Selection of endometrial carcinomas for DNA mismatch repair protein immunohistochemistry using patient age and tumor morphology enhances detection of mismatch repair abnormalities. Am J Surg Pathol 2009;33:925–33.
36. Bansal N, Herzog TJ, Seshan VE, Schiff PB, Burke WM, et al. Uterine carcinosarcomas and grade 3 endometrioid cancers: evidence for distinct tumor behavior. Obstet Gynecol 2008;112:64–70.
37. McCluggage WG. Müllerian adenosarcoma of the female genital tract. Adv Anat Pathol 2010;17:122–29.
38. FIGO Committee in Gynecologic Oncology. FIGO Staging for uterine sarcomas. Int J Gynecol Obstet 2009;104:179.
39. D'Angelo E, Prat J. Uterine sarcomas: a review. Gynecol Oncol 2010;116:131–39.
40. Kempson RL, Hendrickson MR. Smooth muscle, endometrial stromal, and mixed Müllerian tumors of the uterus. Mod Pathol 2000;13: 328–42.
41. McCluggage WG, Ganesan R, Herrington CS. Endometrial stromal sarcomas with extensive endometrioid glandular differentiation: report of a series with emphasis on the potential for misdiagnosis and discussion of the differential diagnosis. Histopathol 2009;54:365–73.
42. Krizova A, Clarke BA, Bernardini MQ, James S, Kalloger SE, et al. Histologic artifacts in abdominal, vaginal, laparoscopic, and robotic hysterectomy specimens: a blinded, retrospective review. Am J Surg Pathol 2011;35:115–26.

8 Pitfalls in diagnosis

Endometrial diagnosis can be difficult. Tissue may frequently resemble the illustrations in a textbook, but there can be a variety of benign changes (artifacts and metaplasias) that make interpretation very difficult. This chapter addresses these changes.

In order to be clinically useful, a diagnosis must convey whether or not an intervention is required by the clinician. Hence, many of the entities discussed below, while important for the pathologist to recognize, may not be deemed critical for inclusion in the final report, and it should be remembered that they may in fact make the report confusing to the clinician.

Artifacts

Artifacts include effects on endometrial tissue due to sampling or fixation, the presence of inactive endometrial tissue, or the presence of nonendometrial tissue that may confuse the diagnosis. It is important to be able to recognize these.

Telescoping

In telescoping artifact, the glands undergo intussusception, giving them a concentric "gland-within-a-gland" appearance (**Figure 8.1**), which should not be construed as glandular crowding.

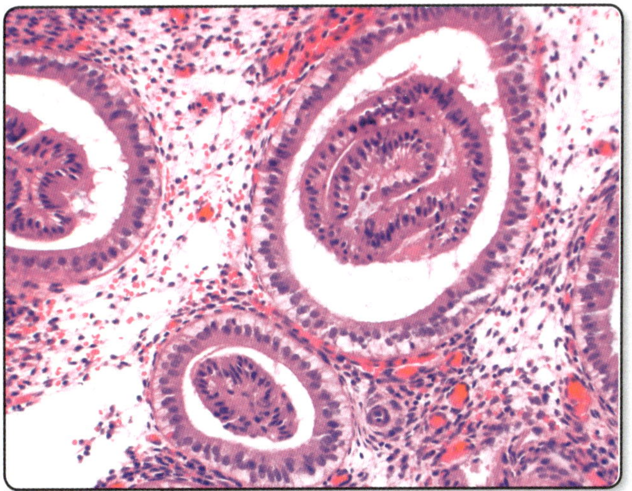

Figure 8.1 Telescoping artifact-glands undergo intussusception. This should not be mistaken for glandular crowding.

Artifactual crowding (squeeze artifact)

Sometimes there appears to be complexity within a single gland, which, particularly on low power, may appear to be crowding. On closer inspection, the lack of crowding of the other glands should assist in distinguishing this artifact from hyperplasia. Crowding artifact is often seen at the edge of a tissue fragment, suggesting trauma to the tissue may be the underlying etiology (**Figure 8.2**).

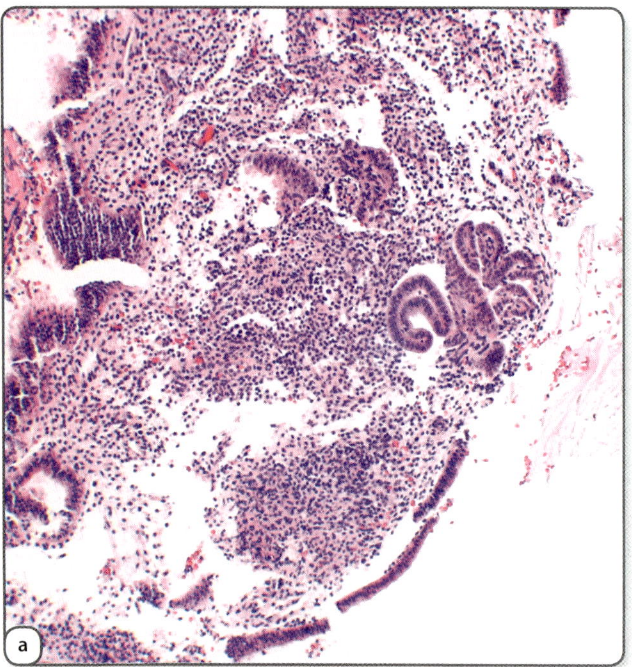

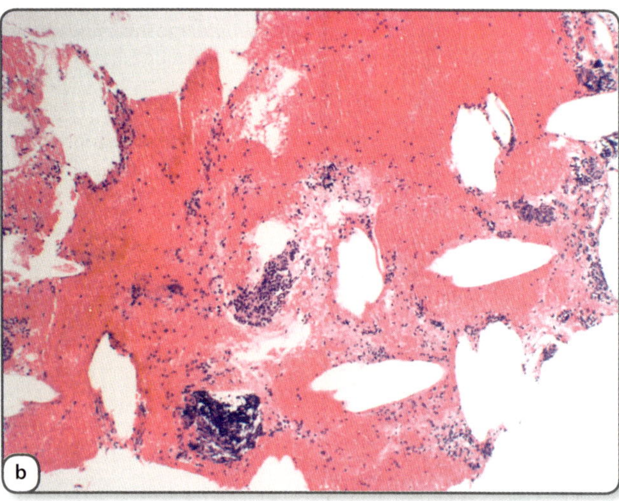

Figure 8.2 Squeeze (crowding) artifact. This is often seen at the edge of a fragment of endometrium (a). Crush or squeezed tissue may also be seen from stuffing too much tissue into a cassette, creating a "waffle" effect, and interfering with interpretation (b).

"Waffle" artifact

If too much tissue is stuffed into a tissue cassette, or sometimes secondary to tissue processing bags that go inside a cassette,[1] a crosshatched waffle shaped pattern may be seen in the tissue from impressions made by the cassette (**Figure 8.3**).

Retraction Artifact

Retraction artifact in the endometrium is usually seen in hysterectomy specimens (**Figure 8.4**), and it should not be mistaken for subnuclear vacuoles. It probably relates to degeneration of the tissue prior to fixation. Within the myometrium, retraction of the myometrium around nests of tumor should not be mistaken for lymphovascular space involvement (see p. 129).

Inactive Fragments

It is important to recognize inactive fragments that are not part of the functional layer of the endometrium, to avoid a false diagnosis of

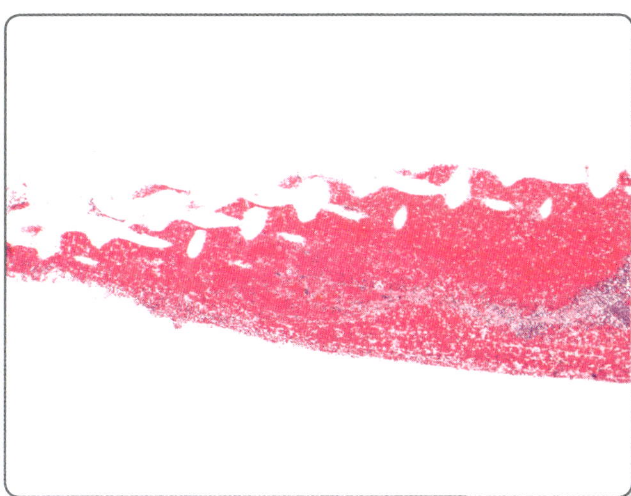

Figure 8.3 Waffle artifact. This endometrial biopsy was stuffed into a cassette, giving the characteristic cross-hatched pattern. Note that the specimen is mostly blood. It was received in long strips in formalin, conforming to the shape of the sampling device. This can be misinterpreted grossly as abundant tissue.

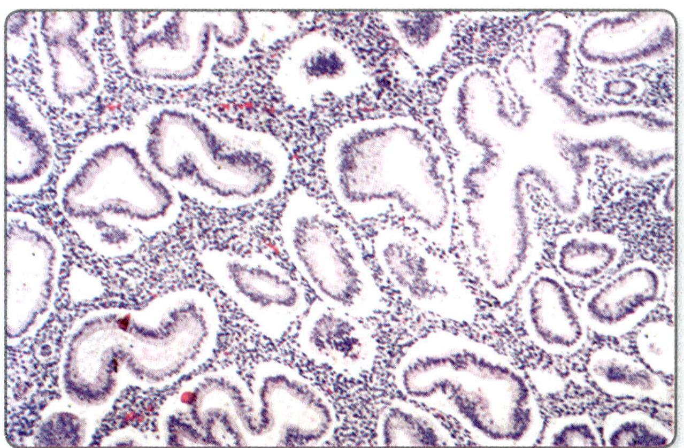

Figure 8.4 Retraction artifact. This is usually seen in hysterectomy specimens, and may relate to a delay in fixation.

inactive or atrophic endometrium when a more concerning lesion is actually present but is unsampled.

Basalis

A clue to the presence of basalis endometrium in curettings is the lack of overlying surface endometrium seen. If full-thickness fragments are obtained, the diagnosis is more easily made. The glands of basalis endometrium show less proliferation than the functionalis, and they are usually weakly proliferative to inactive during the proliferative phase, although they may show secretory features in a secretory endometrium. Prominent blood vessels and lymphoid aggregates may be seen in the hypercellular basophilic stroma (**Figure 8.5**)

Lower Uterine Segment

Lower uterine segment is frequently present in endometrial curettings. The stroma contains more collagen than endometrial stroma and hence appears more eosinophilic and less cellular. The glands appear inactive, and they may show mixed inactive endometrial glands among endocervical glands, or glands with features of both endometrial and endocervical histology. In the absence of endocervical glandular features, the stroma needs to be relied on to make the diagnosis (**Figure 8.6**).

Thermal artifact

Endometrial ablation for persistence of bleeding may have been performed prior to a biopsy or hysterectomy. Depending on the time elapsed since the procedure, changes may include necrosis, foreign

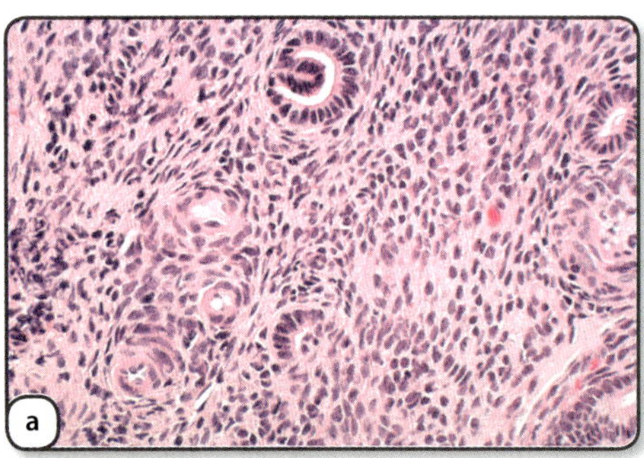

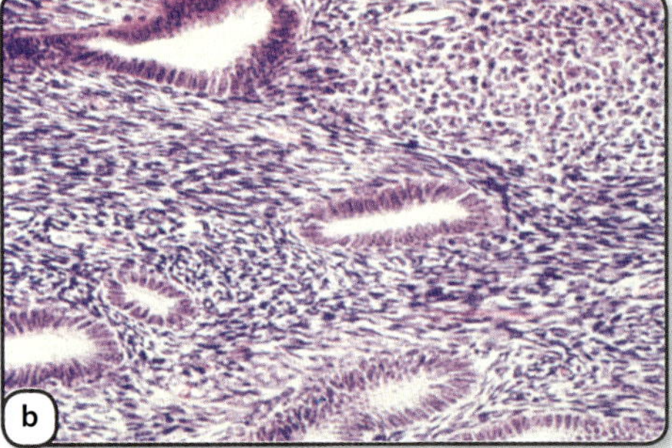

Figure 8.5 Basalis endometrium showing inactive glands in a dense cellular stroma with prominent arterioles (a). Lymphoid aggregates, as seen in the upper right, are a normal finding (b).

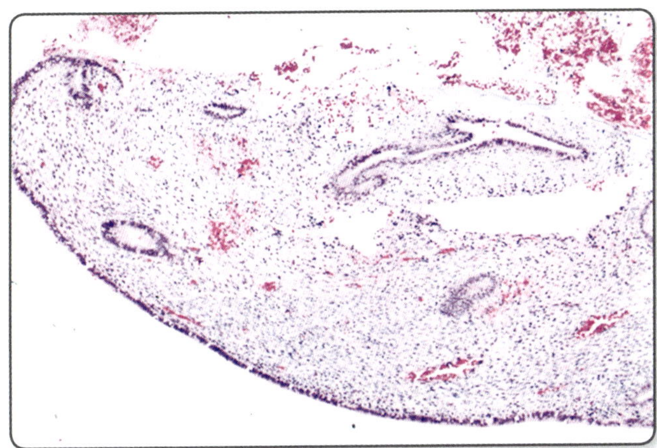

Figure 8.6 Lower uterine segment. The stroma is more eosinophilic than the functionalis stroma, and the glands show mixed endocervical and endometrial features.

body giant cell reaction (granulomatous inflammation), brown or black pigment, thermal artifact on the tissue, hyalinization, and fibrosis[2] (**Figure 8.7**). Residual tissue may remain in failed ablations (**Figure 8.8**). Thermal artifact may also cause vacuolation of endometrial stromal cells, which should not be interpreted as signet ring cells.[3]

Artifactual "lymphvascular space" invasion

To be diagnostic of true lymphovascular space involvement, the tumor emboli usually conform to the shape of the vessels, may be part of an organizing thrombus (**Figure 8.9b**) and the space shows a true endothelial lining. Fixation artifact leading to retraction around a nest of tumor should not be confused with true vascular invasion. Endothelial stains such as CD31 or CD34 on an untrimmed section may be helpful, but are often not in my personal experience. A more difficult distinction is when tumor is very friable, or the endometrium

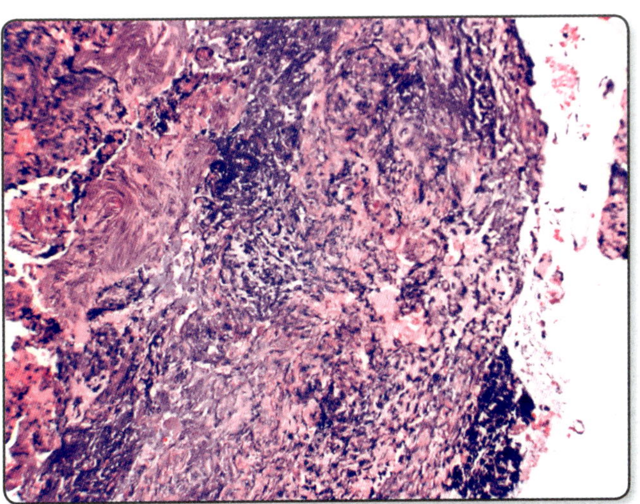

Figure 8.7 Thermal artifact can completely disguise the nature of the tissue, and stretched out nuclei may mimic neoplasia.

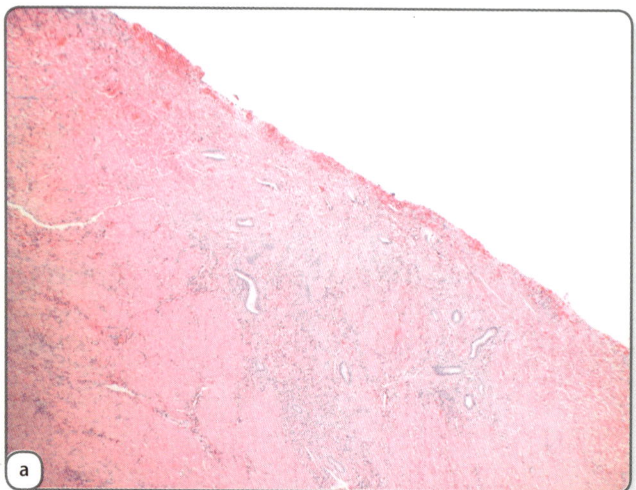

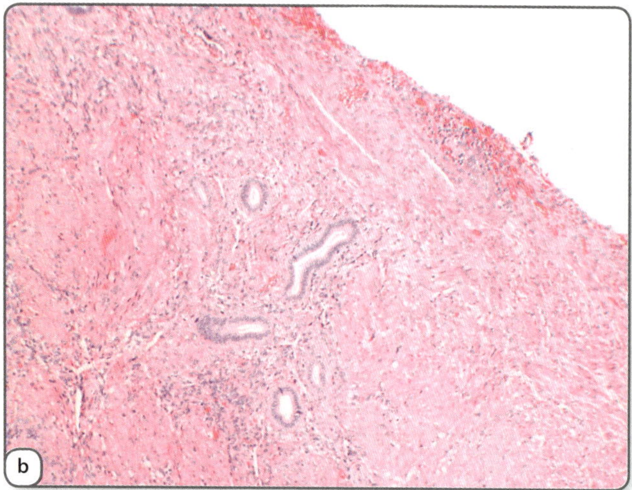

Figure 8.8 Failed endometrial ablation. Note residual endometrium, and hemorrhage on the surface.

is autolyzed and fragments readily, and is seen in vascular spaces, particularly if there has been much uterine manipulation during surgery[4] or during handling in the laboratory. Hysterectomies performed by laparoscopy are particularly prone to pseudoinvasion, possibly due to positive pressure.[2] The tumor may not mold to the shape of the vessels in these cases, but often the pathologist can't tell if this is a true or an artifactual lymphovascular space involvement (**Figure 8.9**).

Lymphvascular space invasion mimicking histiocytes

McKenney et al[5] have described a pattern of lymphvascular space involvement with single cells with abundant cytoplasm, mimicking histiocytes.

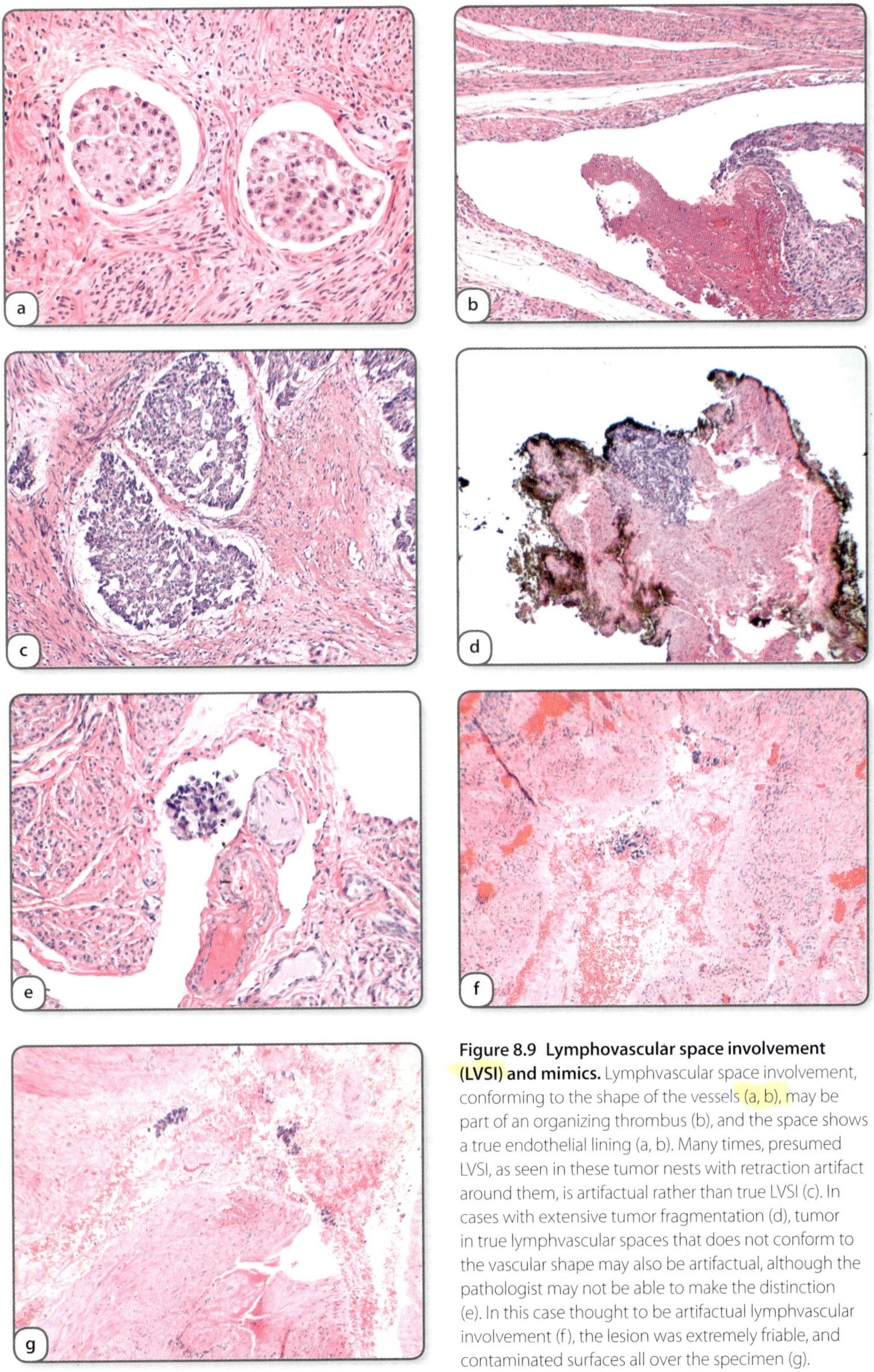

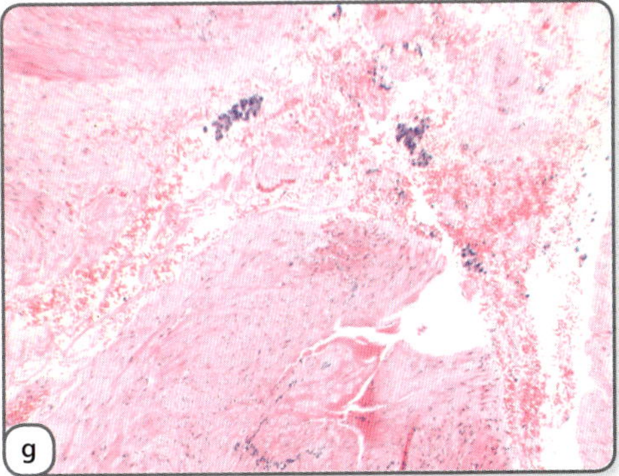

Figure 8.9 Lymphovascular space involvement (LVSI) and mimics. Lymphvascular space involvement, conforming to the shape of the vessels (a, b), may be part of an organizing thrombus (b), and the space shows a true endothelial lining (a, b). Many times, presumed LVSI, as seen in these tumor nests with retraction artifact around them, is artifactual rather than true LVSI (c). In cases with extensive tumor fragmentation (d), tumor in true lymphvascular spaces that does not conform to the vascular shape may also be artifactual, although the pathologist may not be able to make the distinction (e). In this case thought to be artifactual lymphvascular involvement (f), the lesion was extremely friable, and contaminated surfaces all over the specimen (g).

Atypical stromal cells with bizarre nuclei

Atypical stromal cells have been described in vulvovaginal polyps, but they may be seen rarely in endometrial stroma, including endometrial polyps. In one case, these cells were seen adjacent to a polypoid leiomyoma.[6] They were distributed in a bandlike pattern along the surface and showed bizarre nuclei similar to those seen in a symplastic leiomyoma. Some of the cells stained with muscle markers (desmin, smooth muscle actin, h-caldesmon), while others stained with CD10. The authors cautioned that these cells seen in a small endometrial biopsy might erroneously raise the concern of malignancy.

Non-endometrial tissue

A variety of non-endometrial fragments may be seen on endometrial biopsies. Some of them, such as cervical tissue, may fragment off during sampling; hence benign endocervical tissue, tissue with microglandular hyperplasia, or dysplastic squamous epithelium may be seen. Although microglandular hyperplasia may appear as adenocarcinoma on low power, higher power reveals the endocervical and benign nature of the tissue. Dysplastic cervical epithelium is friable, and it is not rare to find it in curettings. This does not mean that the process involves the endometrial cavity. Unless dysplastic squamous epithelium is seen in continuity with endometrium, the pathologist can draw no conclusion about endometrial involvement, which is uncommon.

The presence of adipose tissue in a curetting is uterine perforation until proven otherwise, and the clinician must be notified immediately. By the time this conversation occurs, it is likely that either the clinician is aware of a perforation, or the patient has had no sequelae; however, notification is important. There is an artifact called pseudolipomatosis (**Figure 8.10e–g**), that can be seen in endometrium, with optically clear spaces resembling adipose tissue, however the spaces are more variable in size than adipose tissue. Lack of cohesion and lack of intervening capillaries also may help distinguish pseudolipomatosis from true adipose tissue. It has been postulated that pseudolipomatosis occurs due to introduction of air during suction curettage, or that it may also relate to the chemicals used to sterilize surgical instruments.[7]

Rossi et al[8] described three cases of mesothelial cell strips/clusters in endometrial biopsy, confirmed by WT-1 and calretinin immunostains. The fact that two of the cases also contained adipose tissue is supportive of this representing a uterine perforation.

Another rare artifact is psammoma bodies within a benign endometrium (**Figure 8.10h**), described by Fausett et al.[9] Most of the women in this study were postmenopausal and on hormone replacement therapy and several had endometrial polyps. No malignancies were detected, however it must be remembered that psammoma bodies may reflect a malignancy higher up in the genital tract, i.e. the fallopian tube or ovary.

Rarely, tissue contaminants are seen on slides that are purely contaminants that have occurred during processing of the slides, such as gastric mucosa on a curettage. This can happen during processing of the slide in the water bath, in which case a recut slide will not show the fragment. If the foreign tissue becomes embedded into the tissue block, it will be seen in recut slides as well, and then judgment comes into play on whether or not the tissue fragment belongs to the specimen under review (**Figure 8.10**).

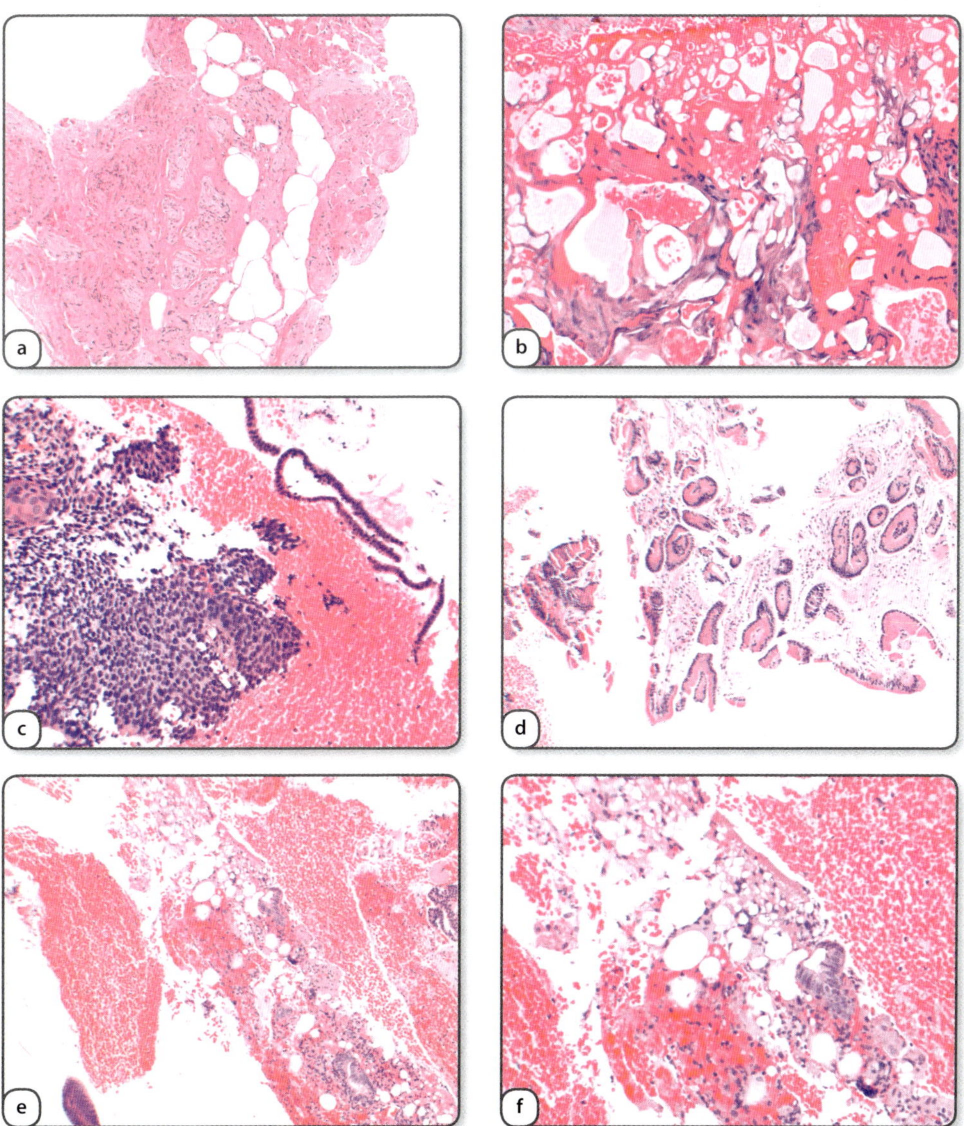

Figure 8.10 Nonendometrial tissue. (a) Adipose tissue, which requires ruling out perforation. (b) Pseudoadipose tissue, here associated with cautery. (c) Fragments of high grade dysplastic squamous epithelium in an endometrial curettage. (d) Fragments of gastric epithelium most likely represent a contaminant ("floater"). (e, f, g) Pseudolipomatosis, showing variability in the size of the vacuoles. (h) Psammoma bodies in an atrophic endometrium.

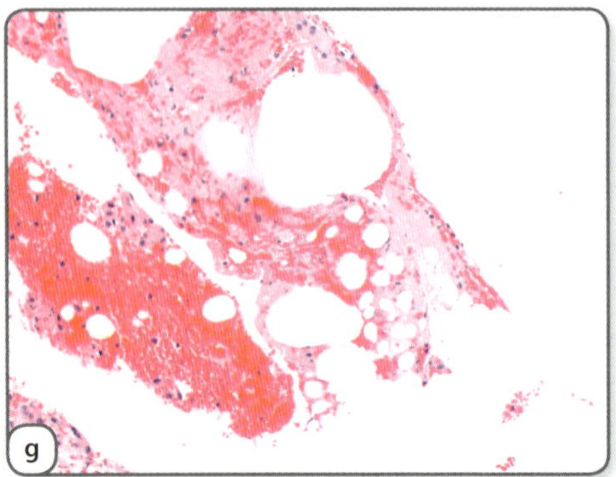

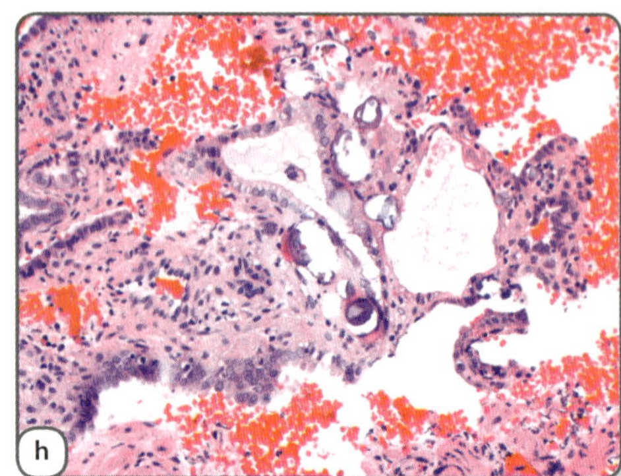

Figure 8.10 Nonendometrial tissue. ***Continued.***

Procedurally and therapeutically related artifacts

With the increasing popularity of and experience with less invasive techniques of hysterectomy increasing, it has come to be known that the additional manipulation the uterus undergoes during some of these procedures increases the risk of a variety of artifacts. Disruption of the endometrium, endomyometrial clefts, contaminants within fallopian tubes, nuclear crush artifact, intravascular inflammatory debris and vascular pseudoinvasion were shown to be significantly more common with total laparoscopic hysterectomies and with the use of a uterine manipulator.[10] In this study there was increased use of immunohistochemistry to type tumors in manipulated uteri, and use of a uterine manipulator increased the likelihood of positive peritoneal washings.[10] The dissemination of malignant cells into the peritoneal cavity is of unknown clinical significance but of concern, and the authors felt that the artifacts potentially hampered pathologic interpretation of prognostic and staging variables.

Uterine artery embolization is utilized to shrink symptomatic leiomyomata, and also to control abnormal bleeding. The endometrium in such cases may be necrotic. In hysterectomy specimens, embolic material may be seen in vessels (**Figure 8.11**). Various materials may be seen, including the more particulate polyvinyl alcohol particles (PVA) particles, and more colloid-appearing trisacryl gelatin spheres.[11]

Taxanes, such as paclitaxel, are chemotherapeutic agents used for ovary, breast, and lung cancers, and may result in the formation of ring mitoses in the endometrium.[2]

Radiation is now rarely used prior to hysterectomy for endometrial carcinoma, but it was previously, and occasionally such specimens will be received. Both neoplastic and non-neoplastic (**Figure 8.12**) glands may show changes in both nuclei and cytoplasm, with enlarged atypical nuclei, prominent nucleoli, and enlarged cytoplasm with vacuolization. Low mitotic activity and no increase in gland-to-stroma ratio may help distinguish radiated non-neoplastic glands.[2]

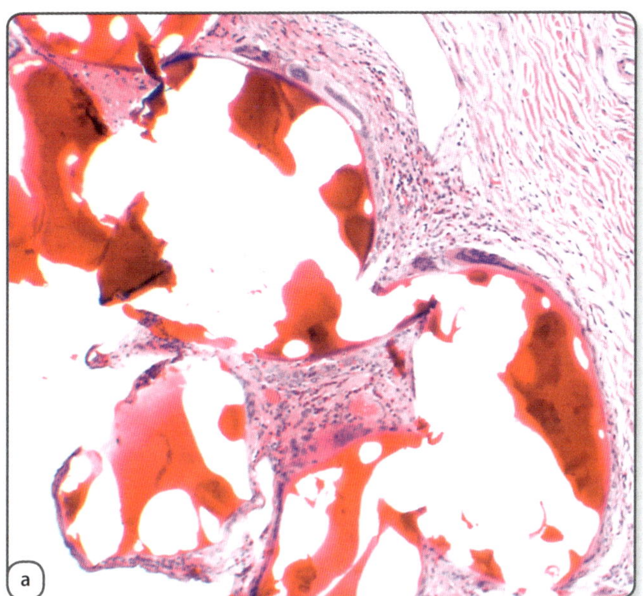

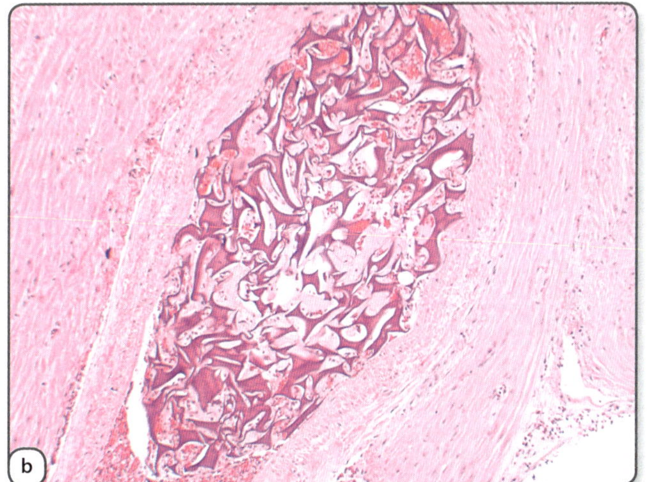

Figure 8.11 Embolic material. A variety of different materials may be observed in myometrial vessels after uterine artery embolization.

Intrauterine devices may be broadly divided into hormonal and non-hormonal. The levonorgestrel-releasing IUD releases, a progestational agent, and the endometrium shows the characteristic glandular atrophy and decidualized stroma associated with progestin use. In addition, perhaps due to the foreign body effect, there is a characteristic surface papillary architecture, with focal ulceration and reactive nuclear atypia.[2]

Metaplasias

Metaplasia is the transformation of one tissue type to another. It may be a normal physiologic process, as in squamous metaplasia of the

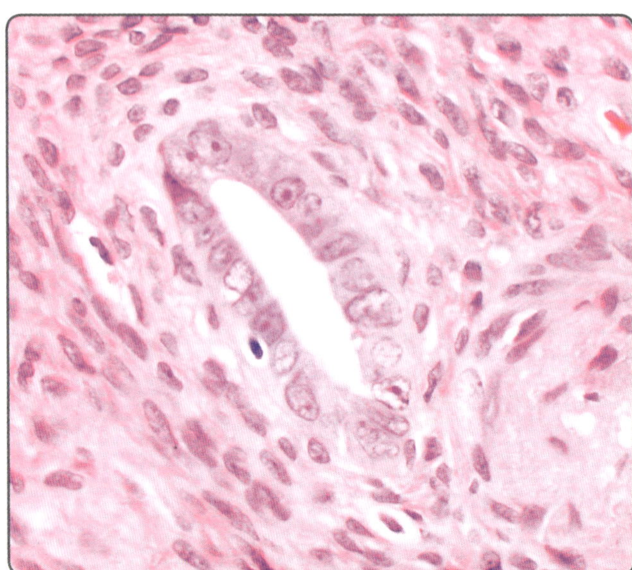

Figure 8.12 Radiation atypia seen in a benign endometrial gland. Note enlarged nuclei with prominent nucleoli.

cervix, or it may be part of an abnormal process. The metaplasias of the endometrium are a group of changes from one benign tissue type to another, usually epithelial, and many are estrogen-related. In and of themselves, they are benign, but they may be associated with a hyperplastic or neoplastic process, or they may make a histologic diagnosis more challenging to render.

Squamous metaplasia

Squamous metaplasia is a frequent finding. It may occur either in the form of balls of immature squamous metaplasia called morules, or as sheets of more mature squamous epithelium (**Figure 8.13**). Squamous metaplasia is thought to be related to unopposed estrogen and frequently is seen in association with hyperplasias and well-differentiated endometrioid carcinoma. The morules may persist in biopsies taken to monitor progestational therapeutic effect on a hyperplasia. In a recent study of preinvasive endometrial lesions, the squamous morules were found to be negative for estrogen and progesterone receptor, and had no or extremely low ki-67 proliferation. PTEN mutations, when present, were detected in both squamous and glandular elements, consistent with common lineage. The authors concluded that the morules are functionally inert, but are associated with and a risk factor for glandular neoplasia.[12] Morules are much more likely to be positive for CD10 than mature squamous metaplasia.[13]

Rarely, the entire endometrium may be replaced by squamous epithelium. A pure squamous cell primary endometrial malignancy is exceptionally rare, and neoplastic squamous epithelium should be considered as possibly of cervical origin first. Rare cases of HPV-positive dysplastic squamous epithelium in the endometrium in association

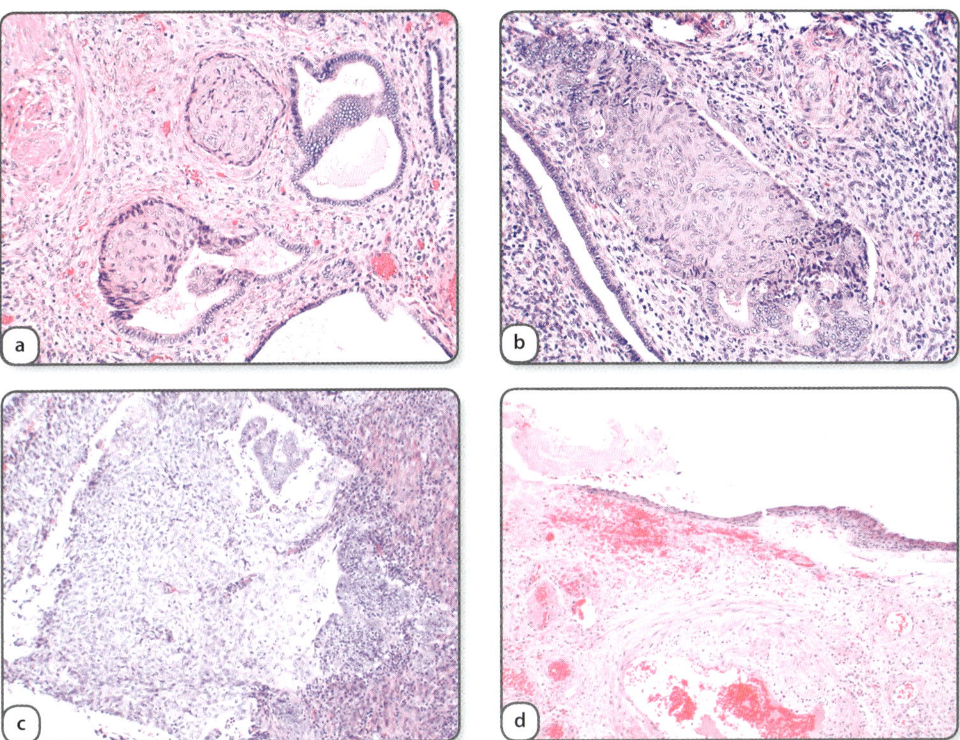

Figure 8.13 Squamous metaplasia. Metaplasia may appear as balls of immature metaplastic squamous epithelium (a, b), or as sheets of more mature squamous epithelium (c). Squamous metaplasia replacing endometrium in a patient with multiple recent curettages (d).

with other HPV-related lesions of the lower genital tract have been described.[14] Benign metaplasia of the endometrium used to be seen many years ago after thermal treatment of postpartum endometritis, leading to a condition that had been termed "ichthyosis uteri". This can also be seen with chronic obstruction of the cervix.[15] In more recent times, squamous metaplasia has been seen in association with uterine artery embolization.[16]

Mucinous metaplasia

Mucinous metaplasia is usually of endocervical type, intestinal (goblet cell) morphology being rare. It can be difficult to distinguish from a well-differentiated mucinous adenocarcinoma, characteristically a histologically bland lesion, particularly on curettings. The differential diagnosis of mucinous metaplasia includes mucinous endometrial adenocarcinoma, mucinous endocervical adenocarcinoma, microglandular hyperplasia of the endocervix, and mucinous neoplasms metastatic to the endometrium,[17] and these may be very difficult to distinguish on curettage specimens, perhaps with the exception of microglandular hyperplasia. Mucinous metaplasia is more often focal, and the presence of more usual endometrial elements, and the finding of endometrial stroma associated with the mucinous glands, may at least serve to help distinguish an endometrial rather than endocervical origin.

Mucinous metaplasia may be associated, among other things, with tamoxifen.[13] It has been suggested that classifying mucinous metaplasia into simple and complex based on architecture is helpful.[13] Simple mucinous metaplasia resembles endocervical glands (**Figure 8.14**). Complex mucinous metaplasia may show infoldings and tufting, or cribriform patterns. Accompanying endometrial hyperplasia may make interpretation even more difficult. The more complex the mucinous metaplasia seen at biopsy, the more likely is a mucinous adenocarcinoma found at hysterectomy;[15,18] however, in the absence of cytologic atypia, mucinous endometrial adenocarcinomas found at subsequent hysterectomy have been shown to be well differentiated, with minimal or no invasion.[18]

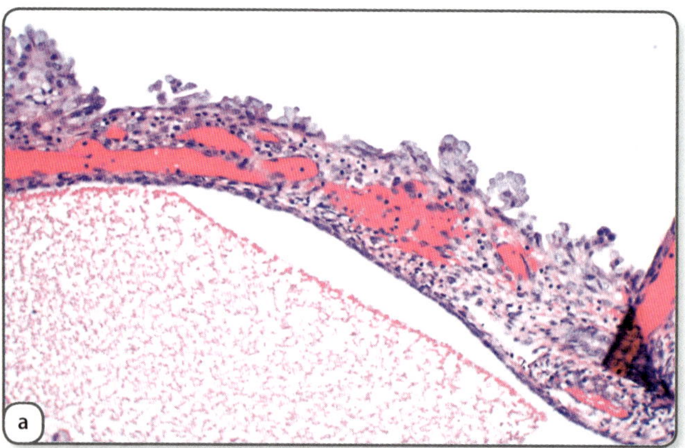

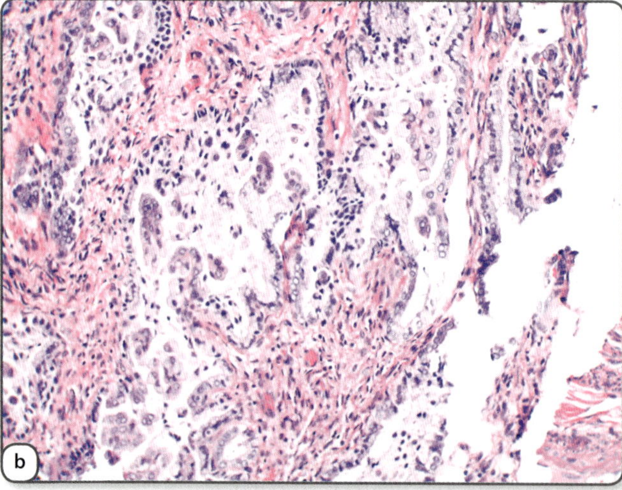

Figure 8.14 Mucinous metaplasia. Endometrial glandular epithelial cells containing mucin. Architecture may be simple (a) or complex (b).

Tubal metaplasia

Tubal metaplasia (**Figure 8.15**) is a common finding in the endometrium. The epithelium resembles fallopian tube (müllerian) epithelium, and consists of the three cell types: ciliated, secretory, and intercalary. If the ciliated component predominates, some call this ciliated metaplasia.[13]

The lesion is thought to relate to unopposed estrogen, and is frequently seen in conjunction with hyperplasia or well-differentiated endometrioid adenocarcinoma, although it may be seen in normal endometrium as well. Although usually seen in simple architectural glands, complex architecture should be evaluated as hyperplasia or carcinoma as appropriate, since the rare ciliated adenocarcinoma also shows no major nuclear atypia, and some cases of complex tubal metaplasia have been shown to have PTEN and K-ras mutations, as seen

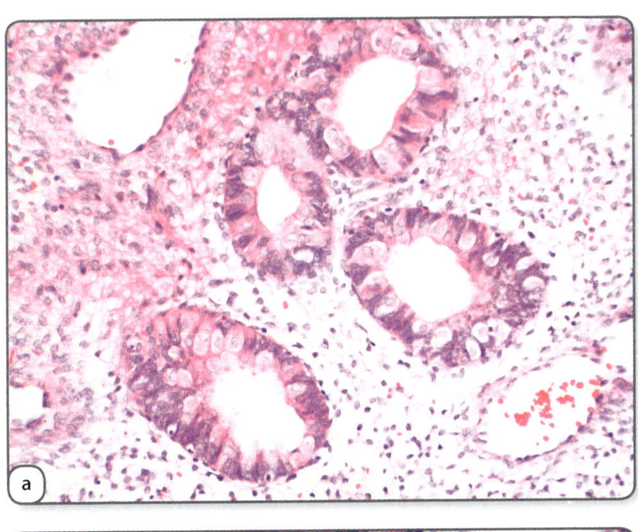

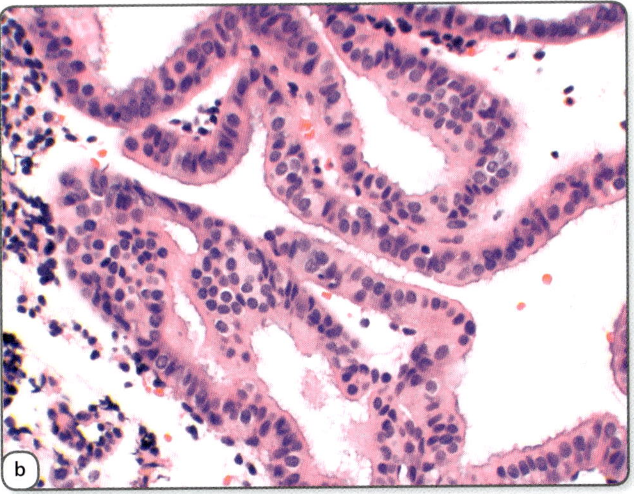

Figure 8.15 Tubal metaplasia. This histologic change resembles fallopian tube epithelium (a), and some of the cells will show cilia (b).

in endometrioid carcinomas.[13] Tubal metaplasia shows focal positivity for p16, minimal Ki-67 index, and weak p53 immunostaining.[13]

Eosinophilic metaplasia

Eosinophilic metaplasia is similar in appearance to tubal metaplasia, but without cilia (**Figure 8.16**). It is associated with hyperplasias and estrogen-related adenocarcinomas, but it may be seen in normal endometrium as well. The cells of eosinophilic metaplasia show no significant atypia or mitotic activity, but they contain abundant eosinophilic cytoplasm. While usually not a problem if of simple architecture, eosinophilic metaplasia often forms papillae. As eosinophilic change can be seen in neoplastic endometrial processes as well, this makes the distinction difficult on some biopsy specimens. Based on staining with the antibody to mucin (MUC5AC) in a high percentage of cases, Moritani et al[19] concluded that eosinophilic change is a subtype of mucinous metaplasia.

Hobnail metaplasia

Hobnail metaplasia is a less common metaplasia, and contains cells resembling hobnails, or corn kernels, with narrower bases and broader tops (**Figure 8.17**). Nicolae et al considered it a reactive change seen after such events as abnormal bleeding or curettage, and related to papillary syncytial change.[13]

Clear cell metaplasia

Clear cell/secretory metaplasia are an uncommon finding. It may represent a hormonal imbalance with transient progestational changes, including vacuolated cells or cells with apocrine snouts, which may be seen in proliferative, hyperplastic or neoplasic endometrium.[13]

Papillary syncytial change

Papillary syncytial change used to be considered a metaplasia, until recognition of the reactive nature of the process (**Figure 8.18**). It is most often seen on the surface of endometrium with associated breakdown. It lacks fibrovascular cores, helping distinguish it from neoplastic papillary processes. It is most likely to be confused with serous carcinomas of the endometrium, or endometrial intraepithelial carcinoma (EIC), the presumed early lesion of serous carcinoma. Papillary syncytial change is strongly positive for p16 and weakly positive for p53, with minimal Ki-67 index, as opposed to serous carcinoma and precursors, which have stronger p53 staining, increased ki-67 index[13] and are likely to have greater nuclear atypia.

Endometrial papillary proliferations devoid of malignant nuclear features

A rare lesion, endometrial papillary proliferations that contain fibrovascular cores but are devoid of nuclear atypia (**Figure 8.19**) may

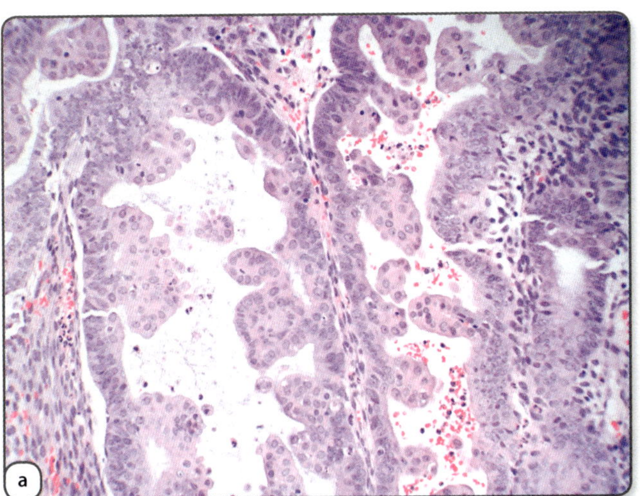

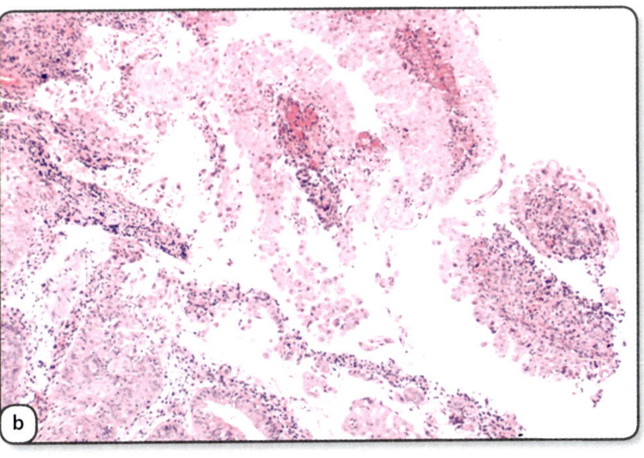

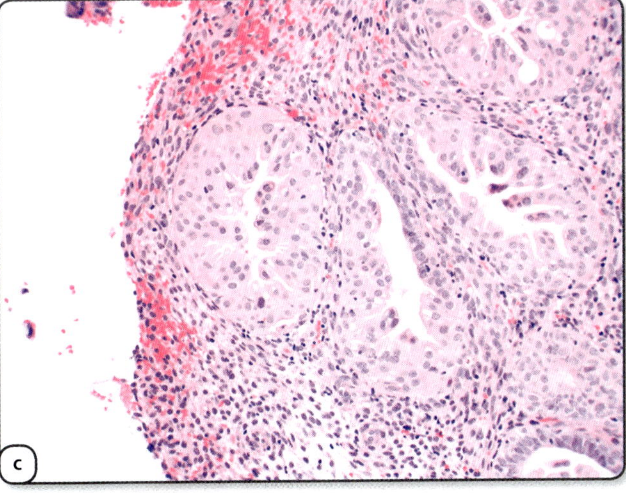

Figure 8.16 Eosinophilic metaplasia may be papillary (a), and may cover the endometrial surface (b). The cells show a large amount of eosinophilic cytoplasm (c).

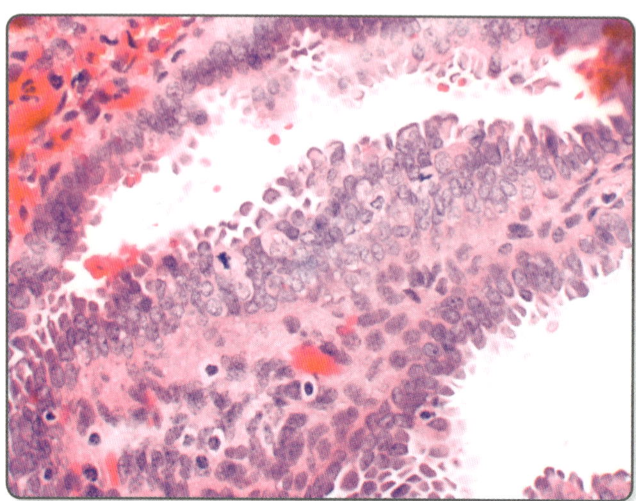

Figure 8.17 Hobnail metaplasia in a sloughing secretory endometrium.

raise the concern of serous carcinoma or its early lesion, endometrial intraepithelial carcinoma (EIC). The limited literature has shown these lesions to be benign in nature.[20] Their architecture may be simple or complex and the lesions may be on the surface or within the endometrium.[20] In cases of difficulty, negative or weak staining of p53 with retention of estrogen receptors should help establish the diagnosis.[15]

Osseous metaplasia

Osseous metaplasia has been thought to be the residua of a prior pregnancy in most cases, but may reflect a postinflammatory or post-traumatic metaplasia, particularly in a nulliparous patient. In a recent study of DNA, Parente et al[21] found that in their series, the DNA in the osseous tissue matched that of the patient, militating against a fetal origin. It can present with infertility[22] (**Figure 8.20**).

Stromal foam cells

Stromal foam cells (**Figure 8.21**) are thought to be associated with unopposed estrogen, and are most commonly seen in association with hyperplasias and well-differentiated endometrioid carcinomas. The cells are seen in the endometrial stroma and consist of large cells with a vacuolated cytoplasm.

Other Stromal metaplasias

Rare cases of cartilaginous, adipose, or smooth muscle metaplasias have been described.[13,23]

Lack of history

Sometimes, a history supplied with a specimen can make all the difference in making a diagnosis, yet it is frequently missing. It behoves

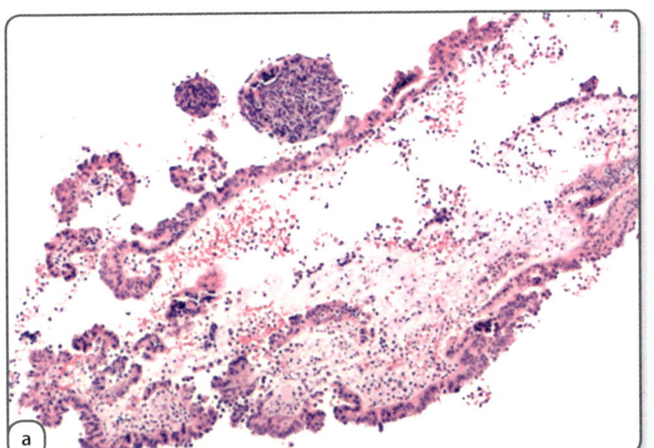

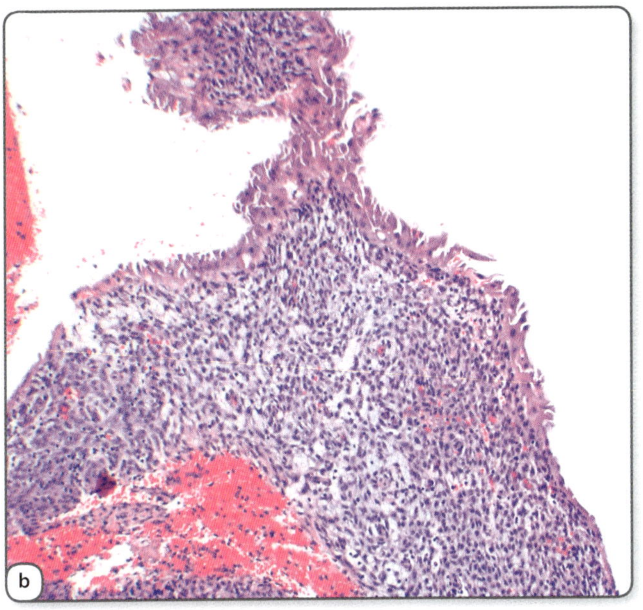

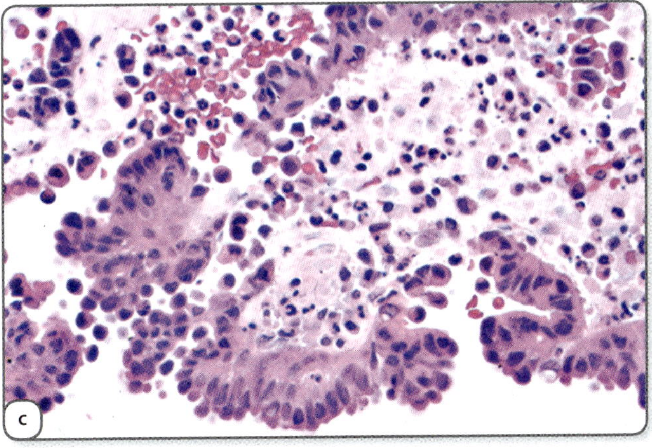

Figure 8.18 Papillary syncytial change is usually associated with breakdown (a), and is a surface change (a, b) marked by papillary structures lacking fibrovascular cores (c).

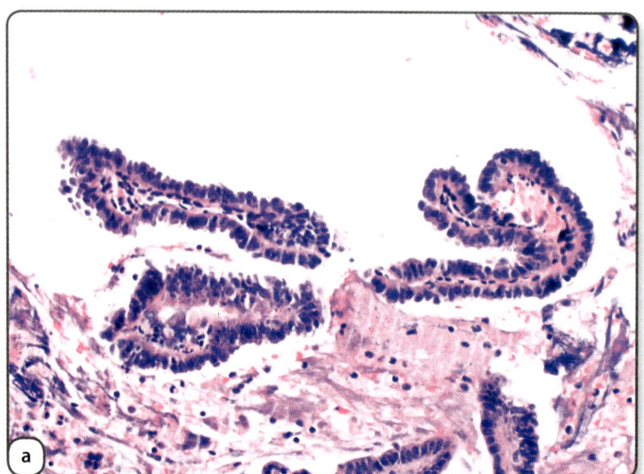

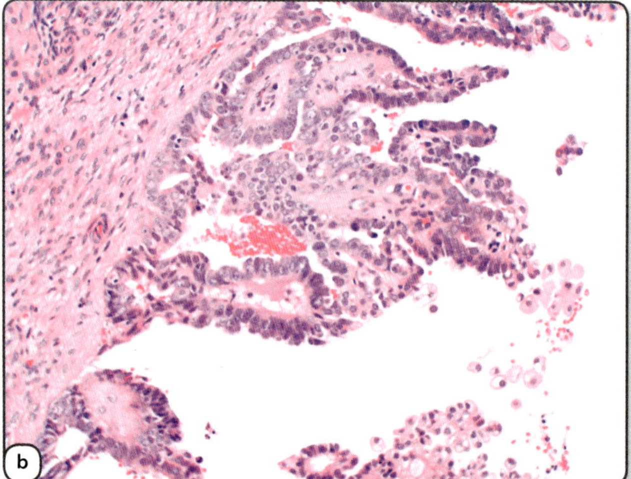

Figure 8.19 Endometrial papillary proliferation devoid of nuclear atypia. These lesions can be confused with serous carcinoma or endometrial intraepithelial carcinoma, but retain estrogen receptors and stain weakly for p53. Note the lack of nuclear atypia (b).

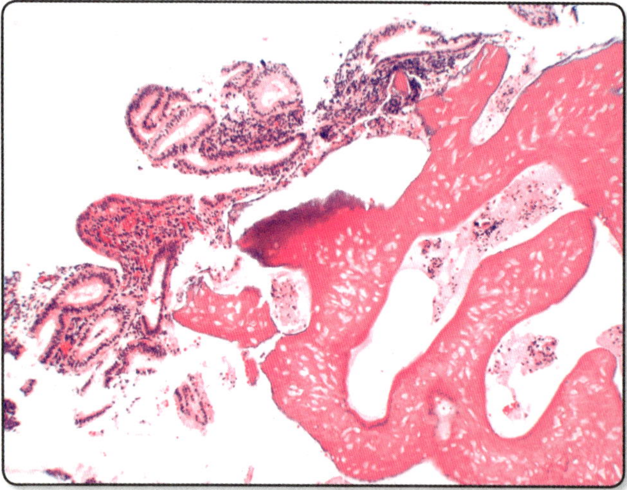

Figure 8.20 Osseous metaplasia. Bony tissue is seen to the right, admixed with endometrial fragments in this curettage specimen.

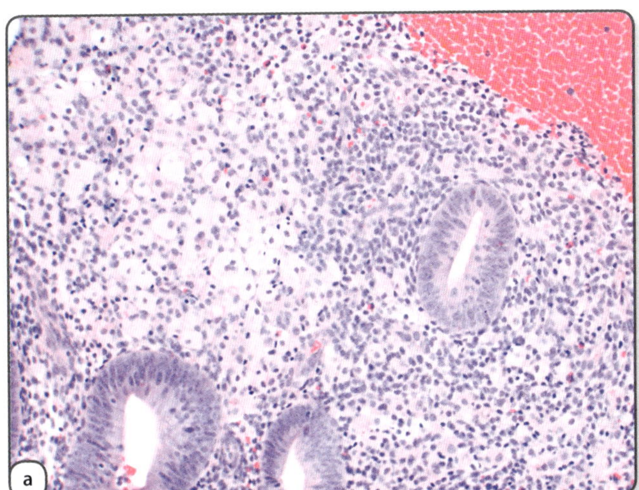

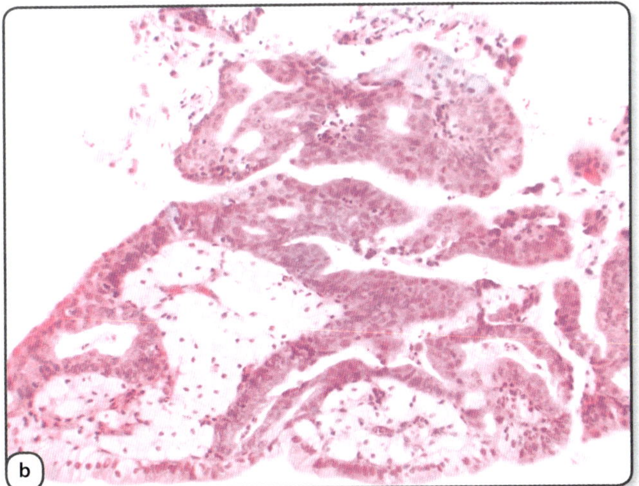

Figure 8.21 Stromal foam cells. A small cluster is seen in endometrial stroma (a). Stromal foam cells may accompany hyperplasia and other metaplasias, such as the mucinous metaplasia seen here (b).

pathologists to make their clinicians aware of the importance of history. Depending on practice setting, this may be easier if the clinicians are known personally, as occurs in a hospital as opposed to a commercial laboratory. Examples of cases where history made the difference are shown in the boxes below.

Case 1

A 50-year-old woman, following a supracervical hysterectomy, underwent a cervical loop electrosurgical excision procedure (LEEP) performed for "menometrorrhagia" and an endocervical polyp. Cervical biopsy showed endometriosis (**Figure 8.22**). While menometrorrhagia per se is not possible after hysterectomy, the patient was experiencing periodic bleeding from the cervical endometriosis, as she still had ovaries.

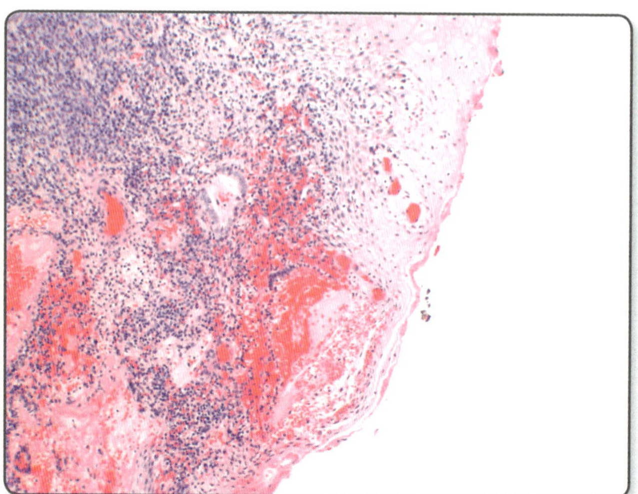

Figure 8.22 Cervical biopsy showing endometriosis.

Case 2

A 34-year-old woman was diagnosed several years prior with atypical endometrial hyperplasia, but was lost to follow-up until recently. She underwent a brief course of exogenous progestin therapy, discontinued 3 weeks prior to the current samples. She underwent a LEEP and endocervical curetting for an abnormal Pap smear as well as an endometrial curettage. The endocervical curettage showed rare atypical papillary endometrial fragments (**Figure 8.23a and b**). Endometrial curettage showed an abundance of papillary endometrium, in a background of hyperplasia ranging from simple to atypical, with focal well-differentiated endometrioid carcinoma (**Figure 8.23c–g**). p53 immunostaining was only focal, and that, combined with the background hyperplasia and age of the patient, mitigates against a diagnosis of a serous carcinoma. The nuclear atypia seen is low, however this may reflect progestational effect, which can mask degree of atypia.

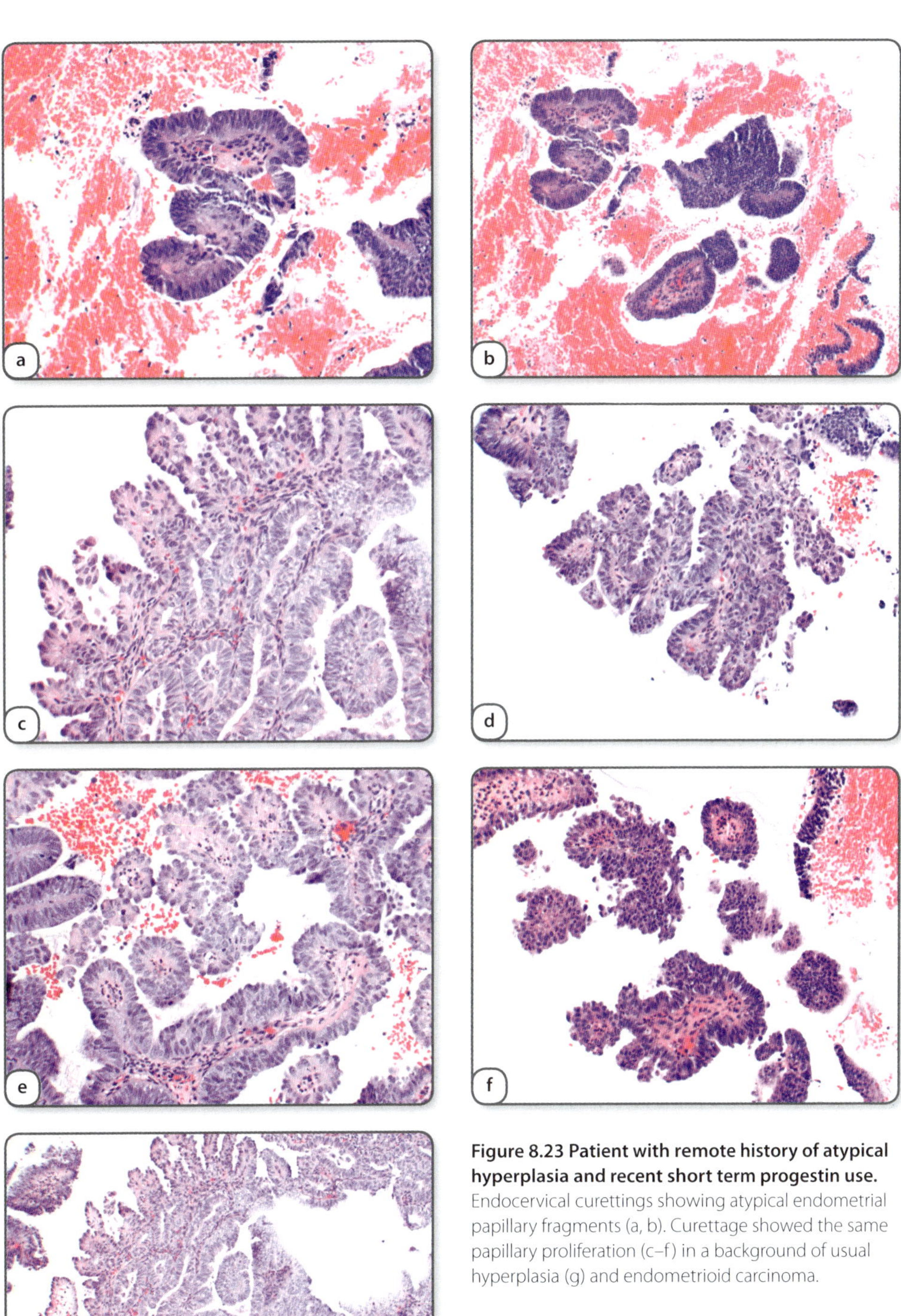

Figure 8.23 Patient with remote history of atypical hyperplasia and recent short term progestin use. Endocervical curettings showing atypical endometrial papillary fragments (a, b). Curettage showed the same papillary proliferation (c–f) in a background of usual hyperplasia (g) and endometrioid carcinoma.

References

1. Niemann, TH, Tranovich JG, DeYoung BR. Biopsy bag artifact. Am J Clin Pathol 1998;110:224–26.
2. Clarke B, McCluggage WG. Iatrogenic lesions and artifacts in gynecological pathology. J. Clin Pathol 2009;62:104–12.
3. McCluggage WG. Miscellaneous disorders involving the endometrium. Semin Diagn Pathol 2010;27:287–310.
4. Folkins AK, Nevadunsky NS, Saleemuddin A, Jarboe Ear, Muto MG, et al. Evaluation of vascular space involvement in endometrial adenocarcinomas: laparoscopic vs abdominal hysterectomies. Mod Pathol 2010;23: 1073–79.
5. McKenney JK, Kong CS, Longacre TA. Endometrial adenocarcinoma associated with subtle lymphvascular space invasion and lymph node metastasis : a histologic pattern mimicking intravascular and sinusoidal histiocytes. Int J Gynecol Pathol 2005;24:73–78.
6. Usubütün A, Karaman N, Ayhan A, Küçükali T. Atypical endometrial stromal cells related with a polypoid leiomyoma with bizarre nuclei. A case report. Int J Gynecol Pathol 2005;24:352–54.
7. Deshmukh-Rane SA, Wu ML. Pseudolipomatosis affects specimens from endometrial biopsies. Am J Clin Pathol 2009;132:74–77.
8. Rossi G, Nannini N, Maccio, L, Cavazza A. Mesothelial cell clusters in endometrial biopsy: another possible source of diagnostic pitfall. Am J Surg Pathol 2010;34:124–25.
9. Fausett MB, Zahn CM, Kendall BS, Barth WH. The significance of psamomma bodies that are found incidentally during endometrial biopsy. Am J Obstet Gynecol. 2002;186:180–83.
10. Krizova A, Clarke BA, Bernardini MQ, James S, Kalloger SE, et al. Histologic artifacts in abdominal, vaginal, laparoscopic, and robotic hysterectomy specimens : a blinded retrospective review. Am J Surg Pathol 2011;35115–26.
11. Maleki Z, Kim HS, Thonse VI et al. Uterine artery embolization with trisacryl gelatin microspheres in women treated for leiomyomas: a clinicopatholgic analysis of alterations in gynecologic surgical specimens. Int J Gynecol Pathol 2010;29:260–68.
12. Lin M, Lomo L, Baak JPA, Eng C, Ince TA, et al. Squamous morules are functionally inert elements of premalignant endometrial neoplasia. Mod Pathol 2009;22:167–74.
13. Nicolae A, Preda O, Nogales FF. Endometrial metaplasias and reactive changes: a spectrum of altered differentiation. J Clin Pathol 2011; 64: 97–106.
14. Sherwood JB, Carlson JA, Gold MA, Chou TY, Isacson C, Talerman A. Squamous metaplasia of the endometrium associated with HPV 6 and 11. Gynecol Oncol 1997; 66:141–45.
15. McCluggage WG. My approach to the interpretation of endometrial biopsies and curettings. J. Clin Pathol 2006;59:801–12.
16. Hameed M, Heller DS, Murphy G. Squamous metaplasia of the endometrium after uterine artery embolization for symptomatic leiomyomata. J Am Assoc Gynecol Laparosc 2002;9:70–72.
17. Hendrickson MR, Kempson RI. Endometrial epithelial metaplasias: proliferations frequently misdiagnosed as adenocarcinoma: report of 89 cases and proposed classification. Am J Surg Pathol 1980;4:525–42.
18. Nucci MR, Prasad CJ, Crum CP, Mutter GL. Mucinous endometrial epithelial proliferations: a morphologic spectrum of changes with diverse clinical significance. Mod Pathol 1999;12:1137–42.
19. Moritani S, Kushima R, Ichihara S, Okabe H, Hattori T, et al. Eosinophilic cell change of the endometrium: a possible relationship to mucinous differentiation. Mod Pathol 2005;18:1243–48.
20. Lehman MB, Hart WR. Simple and complex hyperplastic papillary proliferations of the endometrium: a clinicopathologic study of nine cases of apparently localized papillary lesions with fibrovascular stromal cores and epithelial metaplasia. Am J Surg Pathol. 2001;25:1347–54.
21. Parente RC, Patriarca MT, de Moura Neto RS, de Oliveira MA, Lasmar RB, et al. Genetic analysis of the cause of endometrial osseous metaplasia. Obstet Gynecol 2009; 114:1103–08.
22. Lainas T, Zorzovilis I, Petsas G, Alexopolous E, Lainas G, Ioakimidis T. Osseous metaplasia: case report and review. Fertil Steril 2004;82: 1433–35.
23. Nogales FF, Pavcovich M, Medina MT, Palomino M, Fatty change in the endometrium. Histopathol 1992;20:362–63.

9 Molecular aspects of endometrial disease

Molecular mechanisms of endometrial disease

There have been many advances in our understanding of the mechanisms of abnormal uterine bleeding and endometrial carcinogenesis. This has led to the development of newer diagnostic techniques, and methods of prognostication and therapy. This chapter provides an update on these topics.

Mechanism of bleeding

Understanding of the etiology of abnormal bleeding has been aided by studies that have furthered our knowledge of normal menstrual bleeding. Menses is a very finely tuned process, in which there is universal sloughing of the endometrium. There is an influx of inflammatory mediators and also vascular breakdown, repair, and angiogenesis, which contributes to the cessation of bleeding. Vascular breakdown occurs because of vascular fragility, which is due to increased matrix metalloproteinase (MMP), mediated by the drop in progesterone prior to menses. MMP may also be augmented by the inflammatory mediators released as a result of prostaglandin-induced vasospasm during menses.[1]

It is now thought that when abnormal uterine bleeding occurs because of one of a variety of organic, dysfunctional, and neoplastic processes, it too is due to disturbances of the uterine vasculature and abnormal angiogenesis, with abnormal fragile vessels. Thus, anti-angiogenic agents may be an avenue of therapy in the future.

Mechanisms of carcinogenesis

The concept of two types of endometrial carcinoma with different mechanisms of pathogenesis was put forward by Bokhman in 1983.[2] Type 1 tumors were identified as estrogen related, and hence associated with a variety of clinical indicators of hyperestrogenism, including obesity, anovulation, early menarche and late menopause, infertility, etc. Type 2 tumors, which are predominantly serous, are not estrogen related.[2] It has long been known that serous (type 2) carcinomas of the endometrium are more aggressive than endometrioid (type 1) carcinoma. More recent studies since Bokhman's paper have shown totally different molecular genetic mechanisms for these two neoplasms.

Endometrioid adenocarcinoma

Endometrioid carcinomas are characterized by the loss of the tumor suppressor gene PTEN (phosphatase and tensin homolog). Paired box gene 2 (PAX2), required during embryogenesis, may also be lost. Of interest, immunostaining may reveal loss of these markers in individual glands of normal appearing proliferative endometrium, and this appears to increase with age.[3] This suggests a potential latent and histologically undetectable lesion that may persist through many cycles and potentially progress to carcinoma, along the pathway morphologically described as EIN by some investigators[3] (see Chapter 7) and endometrial hyperplasias by others.[4] Whether the EIN morphologic classification will translate into practical utility among general pathologists in the future remains to be seen, but currently it has not been shown to be any more reproducible than the more familiar WHO classification.[4] Nevertheless, the EIN classification is based on our current understanding of the molecular mechanisms underlying endometrioid carcinoma of the endometrium. PTEN mutations alone, however, do not cause endometrial cancer, as only a small percentage of cases of loss of PTEN function progress to cancer.[3]

Other frequent abnormalities found in endometrioid carcinomas include microsatellite instability, beta-catenin and K-ras mutations. p53 mutations are rare and usually seen in higher grade endometrioid carcinomas if at all, making p53 a potentially useful stain to distinguish endometrioid from serous neoplasms (see p. 101).[4]

Cyclo-oxygenase-2 (COX-2) has been associated with endometrioid carcinoma, and COX-2 enhances the local effect of estrogen. Hence aromatase inhibitors are being evaluated as therapeutic agents for endometrial hyperplasia.[5]

p16 has been shown to stain the squamous as well as the glandular components of endometrioid carcinoma with squamous differentiation,[6] making its utility as a solo stain for distinguishing endometrioid carcinomas from endocervical adenocarcinomas impractical, but it is useful as part of a panel (see p. 101).

Serous carcinoma

Mutations in the tumor suppressor p53 have been noted in both EIC and serous carcinomas, and hence positive p53 staining favors serous over endometrioid differentiation. Even when p53 staining is present in an endometrioid tumor, it is usually weaker and less diffuse than in a serous tumor. In ambiguous cases indeterminate for serous versus grade 3 endometrioid carcinoma, p53 overexpression has been shown to be associated with worse outcome, favoring serous differentiation.[7] p53 mutations have also been noted in some of the cases of endometrial glandular dysplasia, lending support to the theory that this is a precursor lesion of serous carcinoma,[8] although diffuse p53 staining is not generally seen in these lesions.[9] Jarboe et al have suggested that a subset of serous carcinomas arise from a p53 signature seen in histologically normal endometrium, analogous to what has been described in the fallopian tube fimbria.[9] Serous carcinomas have also been shown to have loss of heterozygosity on multiple chromosomes,[10] as well as overexpression of p16, and mutations of human epidermal growth factor receptor 2 (HER2/neu) and alterations of E-cadherin and claudins.[11]

A summary of current knowledge has recently been published by Zheng et al,[11] with a proposed model of endometrial serous carcinogenesis. They propose that the p53 signature is the first occurrence, analogous to what is seen in the fallopian tube, where there is overexpression of p53 but no morphologic change. The first recognizable morphologic change in this model is endometrial glandular dysplasia, progressing to serous EIC, a noninvasive pattern that is seen in the primary site and has been associated with extrauterine disease, and finally to fully developed serous carcinoma. This "missing link" between atrophic or resting endometrium and EIC, i.e. endometrial glandular dysplasia, may be a lesion which if removed can prevent the development of serous carcinoma, although this is not yet proven.

As endometrial dysplasia focal lesions are unlikely to cause bleeding in and of themselves, their diagnosis rests on recognition by the pathologist. Zheng et al[11] recommend the use of a panel of immunostains to distinguish benign from endometrial glandular dysplasia, including p53, IMP3 (seen in some dysplasias), Ki-67, and ER/PR, which would be reduced in dysplasia, but note that there are no formal treatment recommendations at this point.

Clear cell adenocarcinoma

Perhaps because of the rarity of this neoplasm, which is considered a type 2 cancer, very little is known about its molecular pathways at this point.

New diagnostic techniques

Immunohistochemistry

It can sometimes be difficult to distinguish a high-grade endometrioid carcinoma from a serous carcinoma that has minimal or no papillary architecture. With some caveats, a panel of immunohistochemical stains (**Table 9.1** and **Figure 9.1**) can help make the distinction. As treatment and prognosis may differ, this is important.

In general, endometrioid carcinomas may be positive for p53, but it is rarely diffuse and strong, as seen in serous tumors. Low-grade endometrioid carcinomas may be ER/PR positive, but this positivity may not occur in less differentiated tumors. Serous carcinoma is frequently diffusely strongly positive for p53 and ER/PR, and it does

Immunoprofile of endometrial carcinoma		
Immunostain	**Type 1 endometrioid**	**Type 2 serous**
Estrogen receptor	+	-
PTEN	Absence of staining	+
p53	Weak or negative	Diffuse strong positive
p16	Usually negative or weak	Diffuse strong positive

Table 9.1 Immunoprofile of type 1 and type 2 endometrial carcinomas.

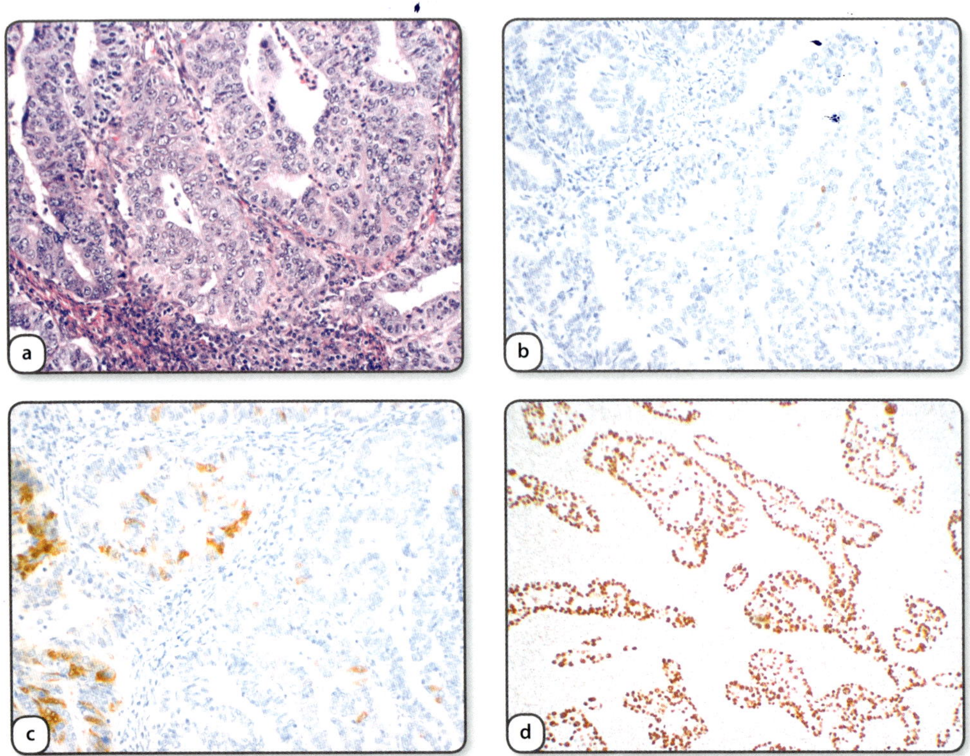

Figure 9.1 Immunohistochemistry applied to endometrial adenocarcinoma. (a) Endometrial adenocarcinoma forming glands, but with very atypical nuclei, raising concern of serous differentiation. The tumor only showed rare p53 positive cells (b), and focal p16 staining (c), consistent with endometrioid differentiation. By contrast, a true serous carcinoma, even if glandular in configuration, is likely to show diffuse strong p53 staining (d).

not show PTEN mutations.[12] p16 is also useful, as it is much more likely to stain a serous carcinoma than an endometrioid tumor.[13]

Although there is loss of PTEN in a large number of endometrioid carcinomas, its presence in histologically normal endometrium precludes its use in diagnosing a carcinoma or atypical hyperplasia or EIN lesion, however it may distinguish one of these from a serous neoplasm.

p63, a p53 homolog, has been shown to stain squamous metaplasia but not morules in the endometrium.[14]

Another area of diagnostic difficulty that can be aided with a panel of immunostains is the distinction of well-differentiated mucinous adenocarcinoma of the endometrium from microglandular hyperplasia of the endocervix. Mucinous adenocarcinoma of the endometrium is more likely to express vimentin, and have a higher Ki-67 proliferation index. Both lesions showed variable staining for ER/PR, and both lack p53 and carcinoembryonic antigen (CEA).[15] Histologic features favoring mucinous adenocarcinoma of endometrium include absence of subnuclear vacuoles, and presence of luminal squamous metaplasia, stromal foam cells, and mitotic activity.[15]

Endometrial stromal tumors are usually h-caldesmon negative while smooth muscle tumors are positive for h-caldesmon,[16] which is helpful as there is some overlap of CD10.

In distinguishing an endometrioid endometrial adenocarcinoma from an endocervical adenocarcinoma, the endometrial primary is likely to stain for vimentin and ER, while the endocervical lesion will be negative for ER/vimentin, and may stain for HPV[17] or p16. However, as mentioned previously, p16 immunostaining may overlap here.[17]

References

1. Ferenczy A. Pathophysiology of endometrial bleeding. Maturitas 2003;45:1–14.
2. Bokhman JV. Two pathogenetic types of endometrial carcinoma Gynecol Oncol 1983;15:10–17.
3. Monte NM, Webster KA, Neuberg D, Dressler GR, Mutter GL. Joint loss of PAX2 and PTEN expression in endometrial precancers and cancer. Cancer Res 2010;70:6225–32.
4. Kurman RJ, McConnell TG. Precursors of endometrial and ovarian carcinoma. Virchows Archiv 2010;456:1–12.
5. Boruban MC, Altundag K, Kilic GS, Blankstein J. From endometrial hyperplasia to endometrial cancer: insight into the biology and possible medical preventive measures. Eur J Cancer Prevention 2008;17:133–88.
6. Chew I, Post MD, Carinelli SG, Campbel S, Di Y, Soslow RA et al. p16 expression in squamous and trophoblastic lesions of the upper female genital tract. Int J Gynecol Pathol 2010;29:5 13–22.
7. Garg K, Leitao MM, Wynveen CA, Sica GL, Shia J, Shi W et al. p53 overexpression in morphologically ambiguous endometrial carcinomas correlates with adverse clinical outcomes. Mod Pathol 2010;23:80–92.
8. Jia L, Liu Y, Yi X, Miron A, Crum CP, Kong B, Zheng W. Endometrial glandular dysplasia with frequent p53 gene mutation: a genetic evidence supporting its precancer nature for endometrial serous carcinoma. Clin Cancer Res. 2008;14:2263–69.
9. Jarboe EA, Pizer ES, Miron A, Monte N, Mutter GL, Crum CP. Evidence for a latent precursor (p53 signature) that may precede serous endometrial intraepithelial carcinoma. Mod Pathol 2009;22:345–50.
10. Arafa M, Somja J, Dehan P, Kridelka F, Goffin F, Boniver J et al. Current concepts in the pathology and epigenetics of endometrial carcinoma. Pathol 2010;42:613–17.
11. Zheng W, Xiang L, Fadare O, Kong B. A proposed model for endometrial serous carcinogenesis. Am J Surg Pathol 2011;35: e1–e14.
12. Sherman ME. Theories of endometrial carcinogenesis: a multidisciplinary approach. Mod Pathol 2000;13:295–308.
13. Alkushi A, Kobel M, Kalloger SE, Gilks CB. High-grade endometrial carcinoma: serous and grade 3 endometrioid carcinomas have different immunophenotypes and outcomes. Int J Gynecol Pathol 2010;29:343–50.

14. Houghton O, McCluggage WG. The expression and diagnostic utility of p63 in the female genital tract. Adv Anat Pathol 2009;16:316–21
15. Qiu W, Mittal K. Comparison of morphologic and immunohistochemical features of cervical microglandular hyperplasia with low-grade mucinous adenocarcinoma of the endometrium. Int J Gynecol Pathol 2003;22:261–65.
16. Nucci MR, O'Connell JT, Huettner P, Cviko A, Sun D, Quade BJ. h-Caldesmon expression effectively distinguishes endometrial stromal tumors from uterine smooth muscle tumors. Am J Surg Pathol 2001; 25:455–463.
17. McCluggage WG. A critical appraisal of the value of immunohistochemistry in the diagnosis of uterine neoplasms. Adv Anat Pathol 2004;11:162–71.

Glossary of terms

Amenorrhea: absence of menses.

Dysfunctional uterine bleeding (DUB): bleeding in the absence of pregnancy, hyperplasia, neoplasia, systemic disease, or organic causes of uterine bleeding. DUB is due to hormonal variations.

Endometrial biopsy: often performed in-office, without need for anesthesia or cervical dilatation. Provides less tissue than curettage, and may miss focal lesions.

Endometrial currettage: performed with a sharp curette, yielding more tissue than in-office biopsy. Usually requires some form of anesthesia, and cervical dilatation.

Endometrial glandular dysplasia: a putative precursor lesion of serous carcinoma.

Endometrial intraepithelial carcinoma (EIC): originally thought of as the precursor lesion of serous carcinoma. Due to its potential to metastasize, now considered early serous carcinoma.

Endometrial intraepithelial neoplasia (EIN): the lesion representing the histologic correlate of the morphometrically defined precursor of endometrioid carcinoma in the EIN classification, defined histologically as volume percent stroma <55%.

Endometrial stripe: image of endometrium seen on transvaginal ultrasound. Can be measured to assess thickness.

Incomplete abortion: passage of some but not all of the products of conception after an early pregnancy loss. If all are passed, it is a complete abortion.

Levels: recuts from a tissue block, trimming and skipping sections in between.

Luteal phase defect: a lag of at least 2 days between the tissue and the clinical menstrual date on two separate occasions.

Menorrhagia: menses that are too heavy.

Metaplasia: change from one tissue type to another.

Metrorrhagia: bleeding between menses.

Missed abortion: demise of the pregnancy without passage of the products. If no fetus is present, this may be a blighted ovum.

Oligomenorrhea: menses occurring too infrequently or decreased in amount.

Polymenorrhea: menses occuring too frequently.

Postmenopausal bleeding: any bleeding of any amount occurring after 1 year of amenorrhea.

Recut: the next recut from a tissue block, without trimming.

Saline sonohysterogram: instillation of saline prior to transvaginal ultrasound, to separate uterine walls, allowing better visualization.

Index

Note: Page numbers with suffix *f* and *t* refer to figures and tables, respectively.

R

S